HERBAL
LOVE
POTIONS

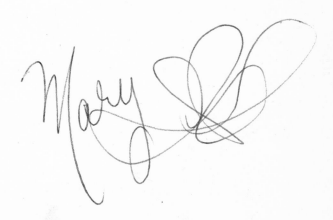

ABOUT THE AUTHORS

WILLIAM H. LEE, D.Sc., R.Ph. is a pharmacist, nutritional researcher, herbalist and author. He is the nutritional columnist for *American Druggist Magazine*.

LYNN LEE, CN is a certified nutritionist, herbalist and Dr. Lee's wife and partner. She is a painter, author and art critic. They have collaborated on a number of articles and books.

HERBAL LOVE POTIONS

An Aphrodisiac Array
of Libido-Lifting Potent Plants

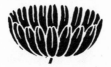

WILLIAM H. LEE, D.Sc., R.Ph.

and

LYNN LEE, CN

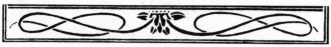

KEATS PUBLISHING, INC. NEW CANAAN, CONNECTICUT

Herbal Love Potions is not intended as medical advice.
Its intent is solely informational and educational.
Please consult a health professional should
the need for one be indicated.

HERBAL LOVE POTIONS

Library of Congress Cataloging-in-Publication Data

Lee, William H.
   Herbal love potions : an aphrodisiac array of libido-lifting
potent plants / by William H. Lee & Lynn Lee.
            p.   cm.
   Includes bibliographical references (p.   ) and index.
   ISBN 0-87983-544-3
   1. Aphrodisiacs. 2. Herbs I. Lee, Lynn, CN II. Title.
RM386.L44   1991
615'.766—dc20   90-23301
                                                    CIP

Printed in the United States of America
Published by Keats Publishing, Inc.
27 Pine Street (Box 876)
New Canaan, Connecticut 06840-0876

CONTENTS

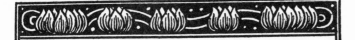

INTRODUCTION
TO
APHRODITE

Yet would I be glad to sleep with golden
Aphrodite. *Homer c. 700 B.C.*

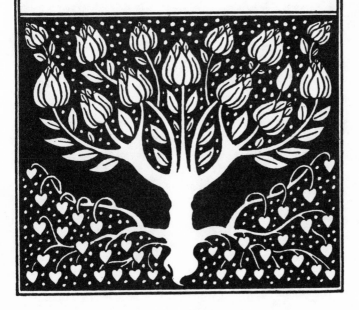

APHRODITE, also known as Kallipygos ("She of the Beautiful Buttocks" or "belle-bottomed") was born full-grown from the sea (*aphros* means "foam"). To the early Romans she was Venus, and to all of us she was and is the symbol of love, a marvelous elixir . . . the all-powerful, all-potent aphrodisiac.

What Is an Aphrodisiac?

According to Webster, it is a substance which excites sexual desire.

That appears to limit aphrodisiacs to a "substance." But some people are turned on by the smell of leather, the smell of apple pie . . . and perhaps the odor of some things that are better not mentioned in this book. Others find the feel of silk on their bodies to be stimulating, even silken flimsies worn by the opposite sex.

Our government recently rounded up a band of poachers accused of the slaughter of hundreds of black bears in the northeastern United States. The poachers were not killing the animals for their meat but for their gall bladders. The gall bladders

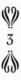

were then to be dried and ground into powder for transport to Asia for sale for as much as $500 an ounce to men who believe that a tiny pinch of the powder can enhance their libido. These men believe that if they devour parts of a powerful animal they will absorb its sexual vitality.

What if the bear's gall bladder fails? They can fall back on a lotion made from camel's hump, a concoction made from tiger's penis or powdered rhinoceros horn.

Legend feeds man's desire for love-power and for outrageous potions. After all, Aphrodite was born from the genitals of the god Uranus who had been dismembered by his son Cronus and thrown into the sea. (Talk about having bad relations in the family!) The story led to the idea that foods from the place of her birth could be the answer for underachieving men with overachieving dreams. Snails, oysters, crabs, seaweed . . . just about anything from her birthplace could make the miracle happen.

If the sea and its creatures don't do the trick, what about things that fly in the air? Some devotees swear by the use of Spanish fly, which is neither Spanish nor a fly.

It is actually a tincture prepared from powdered beetles, also called cantharides.

The result is a powerful blistering agent which can cause an irritation of the male genitalia that can be mistaken for arousal. Delicate female tissue can be badly irritated by this vesicant and either male or female can be badly harmed.

The "Jump of the Month" club had its beginning in the 15th century when Sheik Nefzawi wrote *The Perfumed Garden for the Soul's Delectation*, a compilation of recipes to please every sexual palate. It includes an aphrodisiacal combination of poached sparrow's tongue, 20 almonds, 100 pine nuts washed down with a glass of honey, powdered peacock bones diluted with ass's urine or an apple soaked in armpit sweat. (The last two are less fragrant approaches to sexual combat.)

Most people prefer the herbal approach to improved sexual function. In biblical days, the fabled mandrake root spelled sexual power with a capital S because it resembled the male reproductive organs.

Mandrake may not be found on the shelf of your favorite herb shop but many of the herbs mentioned in this book are available. Of course, sex begins in the upper part of the body and works its way down to the further regions. So a lot depends on you!

This book has been written as an educational and entertaining tool. However, the herbs—while benign in the hands of professional herbalists who are aware of their effects—can be *dangerous* if used in large amounts, in the wrong combinations, or otherwise incorrectly.

If you are taking MAO inhibitors for example, such as certain medicines prescribed for high blood pressure (hypertension) or cardiac disease, some herbs may be harmful. In combination with certain foods (aged cheeses, some wines) and drugs (which herbs are), MAO inhibitors can trigger a sudden and dangerous rise in blood pressure. Where you see this warning, take note and avoid those potions.

There will always be some people who will try anything, even though they don't have the knowledge to use herbs correctly. Let those people be warned to consult an expert.

WHAT ARE
APHRODISIACS

and
Do They Work?

When We send down water upon [the earth],
it quivers, and swells, and puts forth herbs of
every joyous kind.   *The Koran c. 570–632*

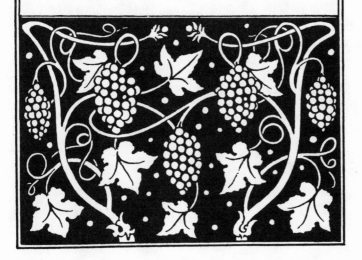

APHRODISIACS are drugs or other agents that arouse or increase sexual desire, named after Aphrodite, the Greek goddess of love and beauty.

Some books differentiate between an aphrodisiac and a love potion. The aphrodisiac is considered to be medicinal in nature, acting through physical means. The love potion is purely magical and is believed to act through occult forces. The former stimulates the sex force in general; the latter directs it to some particular individual. For our purposes, they're both means to a pleasurable end and will be considered synonymous.

Although aphrodisiacs are not the most reliable of medicines, there is too much physical evidence to say they do not exist.

There was a prescription drug called Andro-Medicone which was sold until the 1960s. It was used to increase potency and contained yohimbine hydrochloride and strychnine. So even modern medicine considered the aphrodisiac entirely possible.

Why such a vast panorama of herbs and combinations of herbs and foods?

Because we are all individuals. What will work wonderfully for one person may work just a little for someone else and not at all for a third person. Trial and error is the only answer when it comes to the sexual act which is a form of cooperation between the mind and the body.

Whatever turns you on . . . is an aphrodisiac for you!

Research Shows Some Herbals Do Work

Most scientists place plant-based aphrodisiacs at the fringe of credibility. But one plant preparation in particular called yohimbine, a substance derived from the bark of an African evergreen tree, was tested for its activity at Stanford University and was called a "true aphrodisiac."

Science Digest heralded it as a "cure for impotence." *Time* Magazine said it "has been touted for years as an aphrodisiac."

According to Stanford scientists, in experiments with rats, it increased arousal in sexually experienced male rats, felicitated copulation in sexually naive males, and induced sexual activity in male rats which were previously sexually inactive.

In research done by Drs. Morales and

Surrige of Queen's University in Kingston, Ontario, yohimbine caused sexual arousal and erection by increasing the flow of blood directly to the organ.

(Anyone suffering from heart disease, kidney problems or diabetes should not use yohimbine, nor should it be used in combination with amphetamines or other stimulant drugs. Also, avoid tyramine-containing foods for 12 hours before and after using yohimbine. Those foods include chocolate, cheese, bananas, pineapple, sherry wine, sauerkraut, etc. A combination of certain foods and yohimbine can cause a dangerous rise in blood pressure.)

Nobody said that increasing your sexual ability was not without some risk. Every year some 300 people die in Japan from eating fish. Not any fish, the fish called fugu. Why? Fugu is considered very stimulating to the sexual ability. The problem is that the portion of the fish that is aphrodisiacal in nature is in close proximity to an area that is deadly. If the chef, who has to train for three years before preparing the fish for people's consumption, happens to make a mistake and include a portion of the poisonous flesh . . . the thrill seeker will never make love again.

The Food and Drug Administration (FDA) does not consider yohimbine to be an aphrodisiac and does not feel it is safe to use. So don't think that you'll be able to find it easily. However, if you do, here's a recipe that can improve its activity and make it a lot safer:

Yohimbine Cocktail

Simmer three to five teaspoons powdered bark in a pint of water.
Put into the water 1,000 mg of vitamin C.
Add honey to taste and sip slowly.

Adding the vitamin C to the solution makes a compound called yohimbine ascorbate. It makes a milder concoction.

You may want to discuss this with your doctor before attempting to treat any sexual dysfunction.

The Fort Lauderdale *Sun-Sentinel*, May 11, 1990, in their Home & Garden section, ran a comprehensive article about "Love Drugs." Evidently, even in Florida, the haven of the elderly and retired, interest in aphrodisiacs is still newsworthy.

It covered the Bantus and tea made from the bangala plant, Native Americans and jimson weed, ginseng and so on. Most of the article was devoted to yohimbine and makes note of the FDA's regulation which prohibits the marketing of any over-the-counter product that makes the following types of claims:

"Improves sexual performance," "improves sexual desire," "helps restore sexual vigor," and "builds virility and sexual potency."

Among the substances officially recognized by the FDA as ineffective are anise, fennel, ginseng, goldenseal, licorice, mandrake, nux vomica, sarsaparilla, yohimbine, and (get this!) vitamins.

Therefore, most herbal purveyors are wary of selling herbs as aphrodisiacs. In fact, even though Stanford University has called yohimbine a true aphrodisiac, if a store sells it as such, they may be exposed to FDA action.

It's true that yohimbine has not yet been subjected to the extensive testing needed to formally establish it as safe and effective. As Mark Blumenthal, executive director of the American Botanical Council in Austin, Texas, has said, "Its relative safety is being debated. It is a potent herb with at least the potential for abuse."

In 1984, *Science* magazine carried the report about yohimbine and the study carried out by Stanford endocrinologist Julian Davidson. It said that laboratory rats given yohimbine had increased sexual arousal. Not only did it increase the sexual activity of experienced males, but it induced sexual activity in previously inactive ones!

Yohimbine is derived from the bark of *Corynanthe yohimbé*, an evergreen tree native to Cameroon. For many centuries it has been used as an anesthetic and potent aphrodisiac in Africa and the West Indies. In 1968, the first scientifically credible evaluation of yohimbine in the United States was made by a Phoenix physician Dr. W.W. Miller.

He used a prescription drug called Afrodex which was based on yohimbine. The results, in the words of one commentator, were quite spectacular.

Twenty-one patients took a placebo for four weeks, then Afrodex for four weeks. Another group of men took the same pills in reverse order. The test was double-blind;

neither subjects nor experimenters knew who was getting Afrodex.

Before the study, the patients in the first group reported three erections a week and three orgasms. After four weeks on the placebo (a pill that resembled the Afrodex in shape and taste but had no active ingredients) they reported 11 erections and 8 orgasms weekly, perhaps confirmation of the power of suggestion. But after a month on Afrodex, the same men reported a prodigious 49 weekly erections and 23 orgasms.

The men in the second group reported even better results.

That was in 1968. Why didn't you hear about it? America is very tight-lipped when it comes to sex. Murder, rape, violence are reported in every medium but an aid to sexual pleasure is buried in an obscure journal.

Ginseng, prized as a near panacea for a variety of illnesses, is also highly valued as a treatment for impotence. History shows that it was used to pep up fading virility by Chinese men for thousands of years. Men who have seen many springs and summers take ginseng regularly and are able to satisfy their romantic desires as they did when they were younger.

The herb, particularly the Manchurian variety, has a beneficial effect on sexual and other glands, increasing their hormone-producing activity. The increase of these various hormones is believed responsible for the rejuvenating effect claimed by Chinese physicians who accept the claims as valid.

P.M. Kourenoff, in his book *Oriental Health Remedies*, writes: "Asked by the author of the Chinese-Tibetan remedies which herb he considered to be best for the treatment of sexual impotence, Dr. S.N. Chernych of San Francisco said that ginseng successfully cured patients of this problem *even though it is one of the most difficult disorders to treat.*"

Ginseng does not appear to stimulate the sex glands into unnatural activity. Indeed, it is a restorer of the normally healthy sexual function that has become "weary."

When ginseng was given to stressed-out mice in laboratory experiments, researchers found that the animals were protected from the sexual deterioration that usually accompanies stress. Their conclusion: they had examined some of the pharmacological actions of ginseng and some of the folkloric medicinal values of the plant can indeed be explained by modern science.

Pharmacologist Dr. J. Carr of the University of Maryland believes that the discovery of the chemical constituents of ginseng holds exciting possibilities in the areas of enhancing mental and physical abilities.

Therefore, for lack of virility and energy, fatigue, mental and physical exhaustion, we offer you:

Ginseng Tea
Use one-half teaspoon cut root per cup of water.
Boil for one minute.
Strain and drink two cups with meals or take two to three capsules daily with water.

HOW TO BREW
YOUR OWN
LOVE POTIONS

As herbs and trees bring forth fruit and flour-
ish in May, in likewise every lusty heart that
is in any manner a lover, springeth and
flourisheth in lusty deeds.

Sir Thomas Malory d. 1471

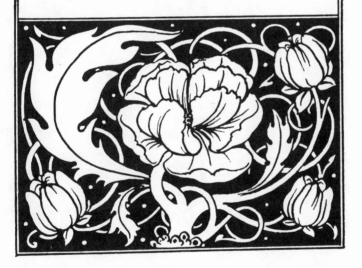

IN OUR contemporary culture where herbalism is often equated with witch-craft, few people are familiar with the age-old terms used for the brewing of herbs, roots and spices. Here's an explanation of the ones you'll see in this book:

Infusion — An infusion is very simply a tea. Sometimes it's referred to as a *tisane*. The traditional method of making an infusion is to place about one ounce of the dried herb in a crock or earthen pot, then pour about one pint of boiling hot water over it.

Cover the pot so the tea can steep for about 10 minutes. Then strain the liquid. The usual dosage for an infusion is to drink about one third of the mixture then, setting aside the rest for doses later in the day or the next morning, depending upon the recipe for the particular remedy.

Often infusions will taste too strong for our palates (made wimpy by so many sweet-eners and sodium), so you can dilute it further if you wish. You can also add honey or juice to make it more palatable.

Infusions or tisanes are usually made from the flowers, berries and leaves of plants.

21

Decoction—Decoctions are generally made from the roots and barks of trees or other plants. The idea is to heat the root or woody substance in water in order to extract the plant's beneficial essence.

The usual strength is about one ounce of the herb to one and a half pints of water. Simmer the herb and water in a pan for about 15 minutes. At this point the liquid will be reduced to approximately a pint (as in the infusion above). Dilute and flavor as you wish.

Elixir—This is another medicinal form of herbs, which usually has an alcohol base and is often sweetened to make it more palatable. It's sometimes called a tonic.

Extract—The herb or plant is treated with alcohol and then the preparation is evaporated.

Tincture—This can be water- or alcohol-based, and traditionally contains about 10 to 20 percent of the medicinal herb in this solution. It's more diluted than an extract.

Electuary—Here the herbs or spices are ground and mixed with honey or other syrup to make a paste, which is then applied externally.

Essential oils — These are concentrated extracts of plants, flowers or herbs that can be used for fragrant baths or in massage oils to be applied all over the body.

Perfumes — Of course we all know what these are, but it's important to note that natural perfumes are made from the volatile oil of the flower. They can be prepared synthetically as well.

Herbal aphrodisiacs may affect us in ways that medical science has difficulty in measuring. After all, sexual arousal is a subjective thing — different for all of us. There is no one substance that is good for all moods, all persons, at all times and in all places.
Many herbal products appear to be relatively safe, however, they have also not been extensively tested by reputable toxicological laboratories so they should be used with care. Some preparations can make you very sleepy after the sex act. Be careful. Don't drive a car unless you are sure of the action of the herb on your individual physiology.

We are all individuals and will react individually to everything, even aspirin. The following herbs have been designated as having aphrodisiacal activity according to folklore. Sample them wisely, eat smartly, exercise according to your own capacity, resolve stress and make love . . .

GINSENG AND YOHIMBINE

Passion's Partners

Is it not strange that desire should so many years outlive performance?
William Shakespeare 1564–1616

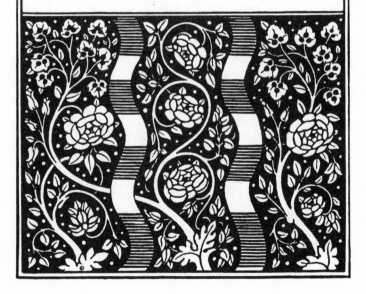

GINSENG / *Panax schinseng*

GINSENG, touted literally for ages as an aid in longevity, has as a side effect the not-unwelcome tendency to boost the libido as well. It's perhaps the most well-known of the aphrodisiacs, and is legally and easily available in many forms.

Orientals extol the virtues of this herb and have used it for a variety of purposes for all of recorded time. Many Orientals, and now an increasing number of Westerners, would not think of letting a day pass without taking one form or another of this substance.

Some of its purported value to humans:

♡ Prolongs life, helps prevent a variety of diseases and disorders including anemia, diabetes, neurasthenia; strengthens the heart, nerves and glands.

♡ Increases and regulates the flow of hormones.

♡ Reduces susceptibility to certain poisons.

♡ Helps people regain strength after an illness.

♡ Improves circulation, aids digestion and provides greater powers of endurance.

♡ And it increases sexual potency!

What a lot to ask from a wrinkled, shriveled herb, the root of the *Panax schinseng* plant.

Ginseng's remedial effects on sexual impotence are not instantaneous. In fact, the Chinese maintain that the herb is not to be classified as an aphrodisiac per se, that is, it does not stimulate activity at once. Indeed, it rebuilds and restores healthy functioning. Therefore it's necessary to use the root regularly over a period of time.

Ginseng is taken in various ways. Some people drink a tea made from the root or chew a bit of the root. Others prefer to take it in powdered form in gelatin capsules or add bulk powder to soup. Still others use it in the form of a tincture or an elixir.

Chinese ritual used to demand that ginseng root be harvested only at midnight during a full moon but now it is grown on ginseng farms (although the wild variety is still considered to be the most potent).

What's in ginseng?

Ginenosides, resin, starch, tannin, aromatic bitters, volatile oils, panacin and unknown factors. One study conducted at the Department of Biochemistry at the Chinese University of Hong Kong concluded that ginseng preparations have been found to increase performance capability in university-age athletes; to improve vitality, mood and the ability to concentrate in middle-aged subjects; and to increase alertness and motor control in the elderly. It seems reasonable that such overall improvements might also improve one's standing in the bedroom olympics.

Try it for whatever reason, it's virtually harmless and nontoxic. The major active ingredients are panaxin, panacene, panaxic acid, phenolase, amylase, schingenin and some vitamins. Taken together they help sharpen the medulla oblongata, stimulate the heart, clear the arteries, relax the nervous system and promote overall good health.

It stands to reason that if you're in good health you'll also enjoy sex more . . . whether or not ginseng contributes to your libido.

That doesn't mean ginseng is not an

aphrodisiac . . . there are, after all, an awful lot of Chinese!

If you're going to go the ginseng route get the best root you can find. A lot of people think that Korean red is the best because the country controls its growth and production. No chemical fertilizer is used and the plants are grown on specially treated soil. After that comes the Korean white. Almost as good but a little cheaper in price.

American Ginseng (*Panax quinquefolius*) is exported to the Orient, mostly to China and the quality is quite good. The Japanese variety is of the lowest quality but if you want to travel third class it's better than nothing.

The Chinese, staunch believers in the health- and pleasure-enhancing properties of herbs, have a fascinating ages-old formula in their pharmacology called Spring Wine. Designed to shift the libido into high gear prior to "pillowing," the recipe also purported to promote longevity and vitality in general.

The herbs were steeped in a strong alcohol solution for a full year before use. (Although some might attribute the bene-

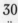

ficial and stimulating effects solely to the alcohol, alcohol has unique uses in Chinese medicine, as opposed to other cultures. In fact, the written ideogram used to form the words *medical* and *doctor* is the symbol for wine.)

In this concoction, the alcohol not only extracted, absorbed and preserved the active ingredients in the herbs, it also facilitated their rapid assimilation from stomach to bloodstream and catalyzed their metabolism in the tissues.

Spring Wine called for, among other unusual ingredients, deerhorn shavings and resin from the antlers, *Panax schinseng* (Ginseng), *Hippocampus coronatus*, *Homo sapiens* and *Equus asinus chinensis*. That's right: powered jackass and human being were part of this mysterious ancient mixture.

Sorry, we can't reveal the exact formula, even if you could come up with the bizarre ingredients. But ginseng was a major part of this passion potion, so here's how to use it:

The root is bitter but if you don't mind the taste, take one inch or so, about the thickness of a lead pencil, and chew on it. After about 10 minutes lay it aside like the chewing gum you stuck on the bedpost. It's good for two or three more sessions before it's used up.

Or, take some of the shaved root, about one teaspoonful to a pint of water, and let it boil for 10 minutes. Strain and sip it the way you sip tea. Hold the brew in your mouth so it can be well mixed with saliva.

Or, use powdered root, one-half teaspoon to a cup of hot water. Sip and hold the brew in your mouth before swallowing.

Or, buy capsules of ginseng in the health food store. Don't swallow them but open the capsule and dump the contents into a cup of water. Add a bit of honey and enjoy.

You can also buy Shaosing wine and take a slug or two daily for your ginseng fix.

YOHIMBINE / *Coryranthe yohimbé*

Yohimbe is both a central nervous system stimulant and a mild hallucinogen. It also inhibits the manufacture of serotonin in the brain. Serotonin is a neurotransmitter that has a calming action upon the body.

The active ingredients are yohimbine,

yohimbiline, and ajmaline, all indole-based alkaloids. The basic alkaloid yohimbine can also be present in the bark as the hydrochloride. In this form it is more easily assimilated through the mucous membrane of the mouth. If it is not present as the hydrochloride it must react with the hydrochloric acid in the stomach in order to be assimilated into the body.

The Bantu-speaking tribes have a long tradition of using the inner shaving of the bark as both a stimulant and an aphrodisiac.

Yohimbine should not be used with MAO inhibitors.

Grandma's Tea Was Never Like This

Here are some other popular aphrodisiac preparations and teas you can make from herbs found easily in your health food store or local herb shop as a prelude to passion.

Stinging Nettle Tea

Use one teaspoon of herb per three to
eight cups of water.
Heat for three to five minutes, but do
not boil.
Strain and drink throughout the day.

Borage Tea

Use one teaspoon per each two cups of
hot water
Do not boil.
Drink throughout the day.

SAW-PALMETTO / *Sevenoa serrulata*

Some herbs appear to zero in on the genitals. One such herb is the saw-palmetto, a
low, shrubby plant found growing in dense
stands along the Atlantic coast in Florida,
Georgia, South Carolina and coastal Texas.
The berries are dark purple to black and
ripen from October to December.

Tea made from the ripe berries was popular with American Indians and we know
what straight arrows they were.

Saw-palmetto Tea

Steep one teaspoon of dried berries
in one cup of hot water.
Take one to two cups a day.

If you prefer, crush and grind the dried berries into a powder and put the powder into capsules. An alcoholic tincture is also available at some herb shops. Try 30 drops once or twice a day.

LICORICE / *Glycyrrhiza glabra*

This is one of the most frequently pre-scribed herbs in China and is no stranger to people in the United States. However, what we think we taste in licorice candy is not licorice at all, but star anise. Licorice contains, as one of the many medicinal ingre-dients, certain estrogenic substances which may account for its value as an aphrodis-iac and sexual stimulant. A combination of licorice root, milk and honey is frequently prescribed in China as a marital aid. Ex-cessive amounts of licorice have been known to raise blood pressure and have a laxative effect among other things so don't overdo.

Interestingly enough, an archaic term for lecherous was *lickerish*.

SARSAPARILLA / *Smilax officinalis*

Sarsaparilla is the dried root of a genus of climbing or trailing vines native to tropical America. On August 11, 1946, the *New York Times* carried the story about the isolation of the male hormone, testosterone, from this herb.

Although loss of potency may be due to many different reasons, chief among them is a lack of sufficient testosterone. The lack of this male hormone can affect the lifestyle of a man, alter his personality, and undermine his confidence in himself. He can develop an inferiority complex as he begins to think that he is less of a man than his fellows. If impotence is a result of his body's inability to supply enough testosterone, then administration of supplemental hormone may restore his sexual power.

According to Adam Gottlieb in *Sex, Drugs and Aphrodisiacs*, the following is considered to be a sure (though perhaps temporary) cure for a lax libido caused by an insufficiency of male hormone:

Sarsaparilla Sipper

Take up to half an ounce of shaved inner
sarsaparilla bark and place in a large pan
with a pint of water.
Simmer for five to ten minutes.
Don't let it boil over—saponins in
the plant cause a lot of foam
so watch the action and lower the heat
if necessary.
Strain the mixture.
Drink a cupful of the liquid
morning and night, swirling the drink
around in your mouth
before swallowing.

Or you can do it the Chinese way,
as follows:

Sarsaparilla with a Kick

Fill a bottle with half sarsaparilla shavings,
one-quarter water and one-quarter vodka.
Let it stand for two weeks,
giving it a good shake once or twice a day.
At the end of the time you'll have a drink
to support your lazy glands.
Take one tablespoon three times a day.

DAMIANA / *Turnera aphrodisiaca*

Damiana has stimulating properties and has been used for nervousness, weakness and exhaustion. It has been recommended as an herb to use for increasing the sperm count in males and to strengthen the ovaries in females. Damiana is also said to help balance hormones in females.

It's used for: bronchitis, emphysema, hormone imbalance, hot flashes, and menopause.

But consider the way an aphrodisiac herbalist looks at damiana. Take:

> One ounce of damiana leaves
> One ounce of saw-palmetto berries
> Grind them to a fine powder.
> Get some 00 gelatin capsules from a friendly pharmacist
> and fill the capsules with the powder.
> Take four capsules a day
> and watch your hopes — and other things —
> rise to your expectations.

Many women in Mexico are apparently not that happy with the lovemaking of their husbands. They've found that a cup or two of damiana tea taken one hour before intercourse helps them get immersed in the sex act. If their husbands are really boring, mixing the damiana tea with saw-palmetto berries on a one-to-one basis can turn Don Lost into Don Juan.

Damiana is a sexual stimulant, circulation booster, diuretic and muscle relaxant. Modern chemistry has identified a number of chemical constituents including an alkaloid damianin which directly stimulates nerves and the sexual organs. Gary Selden, in his book *Aphrodisia* published in 1979, mentions the effect on bulls and stallions and writes about a colleague who drank two cups a day and enjoyed three orgasms a night—at age 69—with a young lover. According to Gary, he sampled the potion himself and reported an increase in his "lust level."

The herb was known and used by the ancient Aztecs as a tonic and a cure for impotence. It grows in desert areas of Texas, Mexico and Africa.

The small shrub has ovate leaves that are broadest toward the top end. The leaves are smooth and pale green. The flowers are yellow and have an aromatic smell with a bitter taste.

For the guy with a heavy date tonight who wants to just put together a love potion and jump into the sack, here's the way to do it:

Damiana Tea

Take two heaping tablespoons of dried leaves and put them in a pot with 10 ounces of water.
Boil for about five minutes.
Cool, strain and drink.
You'll get about an hour's worth of mild euphoria and significant results.

Note: More than one cup of tea a day or excessive long-term use is not recommended and can cause liver damage.

Or, try this:

Damiana Cordial

Soak one ounce of damiana leaves
in one pint of vodka for five days.
Pour off the liquid, strain and filter
through a conical coffee filter paper.
Soak the remaining alcohol-drenched leaves
in one-quarter pint spring water
for another five days
Pour off the liquids, strain and filter
as before.
Heat the water extract to 160 degrees F.
and add half a cup of honey.
Combine the alcohol extract
and the water/honey extract in a jar
and let stand for one month.
A sediment will form as the mixture clarifies.
Siphon off the clear liquid.
Take one or two glasses of the beverage
at night for the best results.

THE FOOD OF LOVE

It's As Close As Your Kitchen

My vegetable love should grow
Vaster than empires, and more slow.
Andrew Marvell 1621–1678

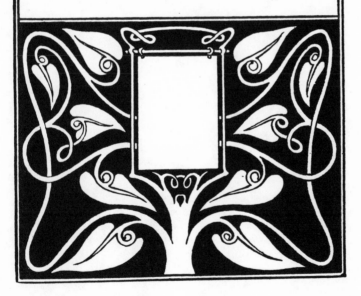

WHEN people think of aphrodisiacs, some think of odd and exotic concoctions from rhinoceros horns, or perhaps poisonous potions made from gnarled roots by gnomes that could kill as easily as inflame desire. The fact is, some of the most well-known herbs, spices and plants with aphrodisiacal qualities are as close as your kitchen cabinets.

Spice Up Your Sex Life

A sex shop in your spice rack? How shocking! But true. The nutmeg in your pumpkin pie, the sage or savory in your stuffing, the saffron on your rice have all been used to spice up love lives as well as appetites throughout recorded history.

CINNAMON / *Cinnamomum cassia*

Chinese cinnamon has a unique taste that has made it one of China's favorite herbs. Although cinnamon is available all over the world, this variety has more powerful tonic action.

It's famed in China as a strengthener

and sexual tonic. Good cinnamon is much richer tasting than the cinnamon used in the West and can be chewed in its raw state.

As a sexual tonic add some cinnamon to suk gok and licorice, or add some cinnamon to suk gok and a bit of ginseng.

Cinnamomum parthenoxylon

This relative of common cinnamon is used in Malaysia for young girls attaining maturity.

PEPPERMINT / *Mentha piperita*

Although this is a common herb and has been used for many other reasons, it's said to be an aphrodisiac in large quantities.

To make an infusion, steep two to three teaspoons of the leaves in one cup of water. Take one to two two cups daily but not for more than one week consecutively.

As a tincture, take 10 to 25 drops depending on your age.

Or take two to three drops on a sugar cube with a glass of hot water.

MARJORAM / *Origanum majorana*

Many symptoms of sexual excitement have been observed in women using this herb.

CLARY SAGE / *Salvia sclarea*

The powdered seed stirred into wine is said to have strong stimulating powers for arousal of the sexual nature.

CLOVE / *Eugenia caryophyllata*

Eating cloves is said to be a sexual adjunct, so, a baked ham with cloves may be an ideal meal for satisfying several appetites.

CORIANDER / *Coriandrum sativum*

The seeds are stimulants. Steep two teaspoons of the dried seeds in one cup of water to make an infusion. Drink one cup daily. As a powder take a quarter teaspoon daily.

SAFFRON / *Crocus sativus*

Caution: Saffron contains a poison that acts on the central nervous system and can cause kidney damage. Ten to 12 grams is a fatal dose for humans.

In spite of its poisonous activity in large doses, saffron has been noted for its aphrodisiac ability.

To make an infusion, steep six to ten stigmas in one-half cup of water. Take one-half to one cup daily.

SAVORY / *Satureja hortensis*

Spices and herbs have been used for centuries on foods to improve the taste, especially in warmer climes where food could go bad easily and taste and smell very offensively. Small amounts were used to disguise the ravages of a lack of refrigeration.

This was one of the herbs used for that purpose. However, it was quickly discovered that *Satureja* had other virtues as well. After feasting on a meal suffused with this herb, people found other areas, besides their stomachs, were stimulated. They began to drink herbal tea without waiting for the first course. And so to the intercourse.

Steep two or three teaspoons of dried herb in one cup of water to use as an infusion. You should take one cup a day a mouthful at a time.

CARDAMOM / *Elettaria cardamomum*

The pod of this plant is considered to be stimulating in the Arab world. The pods can be chewed.

PEPPER

There's red, white, black, capsicum and other forms of pepper. They all have oils which stimulate the heat-sensing nerves of the skin and the mucous membrane. When these oils arrive at the genito-urinary area they create heat and stimulate sensations.

Of course, too much pepper can be overirritating and stimulate the kidneys, thereby interfering with other, more pleasurable pursuits.

NUTMEG / *Myristica fragrans*

This is the nutmeg we all enjoy in an eggnog.

Nutmeg is found in most kitchens, adding its distinctive aroma and flavor to many beloved dishes. It's prepared from the ground seed of the tropical evergreen tree, *Myristica fragrans*. Another spice, mace, is made from the outer covering of the nutmeg.

The seeds were first introduced to Europe by Dutch seamen in the early part of the 17th century and became part of the splendid cookery of all of Europe. The people who settled in America brought the herb with them and it has been part of our cuisine ever since.

However, this common herb also has a "sinister" side to it:

It's a mind-altering drug.

It's a sedative.

It's an aphrodisiac!

Almost all of the herbs mentioned in this book are mind-altering and capable of taking you on a trip, pleasant or unpleasant, safe or dangerous, depending on the amount used.

Nutmeg is no exception, in spite of its harmless reputation.

The substances which make nutmeg more than just a spice are called myristicin, elemecin and safrole. Just where you go when you use this spice depends on the amount ingested. A little bit, say a sprinkle on your rice pudding, can encourage a racy romp but a level teaspoon is enough to take you places you may not care to go.

Want to know where a bad trip can take you?

—One hour of severe nausea and diarrhea
—Heavy, leaden feeling in the extremities
—Lethargic feeling
—Dizziness, flushes, parched mouth and throat, rapid heartbeat, bloodshot eyes, constipation, urinary difficulty, panic and agitation.

In case of extreme overdose even death can result.

A good trip can be amusing, sexy, sensual with a dreamy detached state of mind with which to view your partner and the world. But beware of that innocent bottle of nutmeg sitting so quietly in your spice rack and its dual nature.

What other spices are sitting on the shelf

quietly just waiting for you to make a mistake in the recipe for curried rice or Tandori chicken?

❧ Eat Your Veggies ❧

When Mom told you to eat your fruits and vegetables and you'd grow up to be big and strong, the bedroom was the farthest thing from her mind. But many vegetables have been associated with increased strength and virility through the ages.

For some, the association may have first been made through their suggestive shape (like mushrooms, bananas, plantains, asparagus, or the so-called female fruit, the fig). But now nutritionists are confirming what our randy ancestors knew all along: Many "sex foods" have vital nutrients that can help your love life, as well as give you a long life.

ASPARAGUS / *Asparagus officinalis*

Consider the shape of the asparagus: long, erect, firm to the touch when it is young.

Is it any wonder that the Law of Similars stated that it would be useful as an aphrodisiac?

Asparagus contains asparagine which imparts a particular odor to the urine resembling cat pee. This was another reason for its legendary veneration since cats make violent and loud love in the dark.

Eat your asparagus and make an infusion of asparagus root by soaking several pieces in boiling water for five minutes. Strain and drink two ounces every evening before bedtime for a week.

WILD ASPARAGUS ROOT
Asparagus lucidus

This vital treasure manifests as "all-embracing love."

Raw asparagus root is soft, chewy and sweet to eat. When it's good it has the consistency of a jelly bean.

OKRA / *Hibiscus esulentus*

Picture the okra. Slimy, stiff, gelatinous . . . this uncooked vegetable is considered to be an aphrodisiac in every land where it is eaten. Its usual use is for its nutritional power since it contains important amounts of calcium, phosphorus and iron as well as vitamin A.

Okra is one of the main constituents in Creole dishes and gumbo.

ARTICHOKES / *Cynara scolymus*

Artichokes, prepared the usual way by boiling and then dipping the leaves into a butter sauce, are delicious but not usually exciting to the genitals.

However, try boiling them until the leaves can be removed easily. Then boil them for three minutes in goat's milk. Strain, sprinkle mace and nutmeg on the leaves, add some honey and eat.

This recipe is said to instill lust and fever for love in even the most tranquil of people.

Extracts of the leaves are also used as a sexual stimulant.

SHITAKE MUSHROOMS

These mushrooms are used for a multitude of healing reasons but we will concentrate only on their sexual power.

The molecular formula for vitamin D_2 contained in the shitake mushroom closely resembles that of certain hormones and this may account for the effect it has on sexual strength.

In the case of men, incomplete erection is a common complaint. Blood cannot sufficiently engorge the erectile tissue in the penis to ensure complete erection. This may be a result of disease or stress.

Users claim daily use of shitake can correct this situation and restore full recovery.

Shitake is also said to have a stimulating effect on females, making the nipples redder and the woman more responsive.

TRUFFLES / *Tuber melanosporum*

This underground representative of the aphrodisiacs is better known as truffles. They represent the fruit of a fungus that lives beneath the earth. Trained animals, pigs and dogs mostly, locate them by their smell. A good trained dog is worth a hundred pigs because pigs like truffles even more than people do and tend to eat them once they have been located. Dogs, being man's best friend, content themselves with a pat on the head and an occasional cookie.

The erotic ability of truffles has been researched and proved since the most ancient of times. The early Romans traded gold and jewels for truffles uncovered in Libya since Libyan truffles were more powerful in action and more pleasant in taste. African and Grecian truffles were also in great demand.

The modern kitchen has continued the legend, considering its use to be the height of culinary aphrodisia.

In ancient times, truffles were fed to both men and women since it is inflaming to men and renders women more compliant. Nowadays, since we understand that women want sex and are not merely "compliant," and with the cost of truffles rising daily, it's every man for himself!

DILL / *Anethum graveolens*

Dill seed and herbs are frequently used with other spices to make herbal love potions, but dill is also stimulating when steeped in a cup of boiled water and sipped.

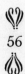

EGGPLANT / *Solanum melongena*

Thomas Jefferson introduced eggplant into America's cuisine but whether or not he knew of its reputation is unknown. It originated in Spain or Africa depending on which book you read.

This deep purple vegetable is a favorite of many peoples, especially cooked in olive oil with Italian cheese.

However, to turn the eggplant into a stimulant it must first be boiled, peeled, and then chopped. Mix with flour, white pepper, cayenne, saffron and milk and simmer for 15 minutes. Then add Italian cheese and a whole lemon.

I've never tried this mixture, preferring eggplant cooked with onions, garlic and brown rice.

GARLIC / *Allium sativum*

Try this but make sure your partner partakes at the same time.

You'll be pleasantly surprised with the results.

Garlic Cloves Amour

Put 15 garlic cloves in a casserole dish.
Add three tablespoons of butter.
Add a teaspoon of corn oil or peanut oil.
Place in the oven and bake at 350 degrees
for 20 minutes.
Add some salt and pepper and
baste them a number of times.
Remove from the oven and eat them like
salted peanuts with a glass of red wine.

CHICK PEAS / *Cicer arietinum*

As a food, chick peas are excellent, supplying nutrient factors as well as fiber.
To turn them into sexual stimulants requires a bit more than just heating them.

Marinated Chick Peas

Juice an onion.
Mix the juice with a tablespoon of honey.
Let the peas stand in this mixture
for eight hours.
Then cook the mixture till boiling,
let simmer for 10 minutes and eat.

ARUGULA OR RUCOLA / *Eruca sativa*

Look for this lettuce in an Italian neighborhood. It has a bittersweet taste and ancient Romans swore by its erectile ability.

You can make a salad and serve it to your mate without his knowledge that it will pick up his amorous approach to your bed.

Mix a few leaves of lettuce with a few leaves of rucola (arugula) and garnish with apple cider vinegar, oil, salt, pepper, sliced garlic and some salted peanuts.

With this salad, some aged cheese and a glass of Chianti . . . you can look forward to an evening of love.

AVOCADO / *Persea americana*

Avocados are storehouses of nutrients with loads of potassium, phosphorus, sulphur, magnesium and other elements. Besides being a good food, the avocado is credited with supplying the energy and desire for sex.

A good diet is considered to be a prerequisite for a good sex life. The avocado stimulates the sexual appetite as it satisfies the physical appetite.

WATERCRESS / *Nasturtium officinale*

Watercress is frequently found on American plates since its delightful green color brightens up any meal. Nutritionally speaking it is a wonderful source of vitamins, minerals and trace elements, however, the seeds of the plant have stimulant and aphrodisiac qualities.

The seeds are placed in water and simmered for 10 to 20 minutes. Then the mixture is strained and used as a tonic tea three times a day.

WATER CHESTNUT / *Torilis japonica*

One man's food is another man's aphrodisiac.

Indians consider the water chestnut to be a panacea for men having difficulty impregnating their wives. The seed is nutritious, containing large amounts of the trace mineral manganese, so it is plausible that making the body healthier will contribute to better sperm production.

In China the water chestnut is considered to be a nutritious food while other areas use it as a substitute for sago.

CELERY / *Apium graveolens*

If you check *Potter Cyclopaedia of Herbs*, the celery you have always eaten as a healthful vegetable also has hidden aphrodisiacal abilities—providing you prepare it in certain ways.

You can't just wash it and chomp it down, then wait for an erection.

Celery Sex Tonic

Put four pieces of celery into a pot
of boiling water.
Let steep for 20 minutes,
then add a chopped clove of garlic,
a sprinkle of black pepper,
a sprinkle of cinnamon and
a dash of nutmeg.
Add a dollop of honey, stir
and drink a shot every three hours.

Then see if sex doesn't go better with celery.

A yellowish oil extracted from the root of the celery can restore sexual potency impaired by illness. Use two drops of the

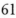

essence on a sugar cube or in a glass of honeyed water twice daily.

LEEKS / *Allium porrum*

Make a decoction in one cup of water.

ONION / *Allium cepa*

Onion juice is said to be able to restore sexual potency which has been impaired by illness.

Onion Extract

Take one teaspoon of onion juice three or four times a day.

Or try:

Soak a chopped onion in one cup of water for two to four days.
Strain.
Take half a cup daily.

LETTUCE / *Lactuca virosa*
Lactuca sativa capitata

What's a good meal to serve as a prelude to a night of passion? Steak? Pasta? Oysters?

No! Try a wild lettuce salad.

Wild lettuce (*Lactuca virosa*) or even common lettuce (*Lactuca sativa capitata*) contains lactucarium, an alkaloid drug.

Why should you be surprised that foods contain drugs? A food is simply an herbal that is called a food by virtue of the fact that it has the name of a fruit or a vegetable. Coffee is a drug and so are tea and cocoa.

But, you just can't serve a lettuce salad the way it comes from the supermarket. Love requires preparation and forethought, and in this case a juicing and drying process, since this aphrodisiac is smoked.

Then again, rabbits eat a lot of lettuce but they don't smoke, so why not try a salad?

When allowed to go to seed, lettuce contains a milky juice that has a mild narcotic effect and promotes feelings of sexual stimulation.

Although leaf lettuce or table lettuce does not contain the fluid, eating lettuce before bedtime can be helpful for those who have difficulty falling asleep.

Aphrodisiacs in your oat bran? Certainly. And here's some other foods you may have handy in your kitchen that will also do the trick.

OATS / *Avena sativa*

The medicinal action of oats is that of a stimulant, nerve-cell nutrient and nerve tonic. Oats are considered valuable as a remedy for strengthening and restoring nerve force to the entire system, with a specific beneficial effect on the generative system.

In China, oats are rated an effective agent in conditions of impotence or sexual debility due to over-indulgence since they are said to produce a tonic effect on the nerve structure of the sexual organs.

Eating oats helps control cholesterol levels but for sexual health it's better to use the fluid extract. Take 15 drops in a small glass of water three times a day between meals.

Hot water speeds its activity for fans of quickies, but in cold water the effect is longer-lasting.

FIG TREE / *Ficus religiosa*

The bark boiled with milk is used as a sexual stimulant. And then there are the figs themselves which are a powerhouse of nutritious energy—sexual and otherwise.

VANILLA

I didn't know this was an aphrodisiac until I began researching this book. Vanilla comes from the fermented unripe fruit of a tropical climbing orchid. Vanilla beans can cause inflammation.

Countess du Barry used it.

Mexican doctors use it.

Mexican Indians mix vanilla with their cocoa.

Steep a pod in some good brandy for three weeks then take a shot—only one—and see!

WALNUT / *Juglans regia*

The English walnut is noted for its nutmeat, however, a decoction of the green shell surrounding the walnut has been recommended for fading virility.

> ## Decoction
> Take four teaspoons of chopped green shells
> in one cup of water.
> Use one cup a day,
> a mouthful at a time.

❦ . . . And Caviar Dreams ❦

Let's pause in this manuscript for a commercial.

There once was a Romanoff czar
Whose sexual tastes were bizarre.
He gave in to his urgin'
To make love to a sturgeon
And so begat royal caviar.

Except it's the other way around. Fish eggs can be very stimulating to anyone's love life. Does caviar belong in a book about herbals? Probably not. But it's a good thing to know about as far as aphrodisiacs go.

We're from the sea. We began in the sea. We carry the sea around with us in our bloodstream so sea elements like fish eggs do something for us. In this case, they nourish our libido.

What makes this food a veritable power-house of love?

In 100 grams of caviar there are 335 mg of bioactive phosphorus ready and eager to be transformed into metabolic activity.

The sturgeon has done all of the work for us, readying the mineral and combining it with other deep sea nutrients for erectile activity.

In *America's Sex and Marriage Problems*, Dr. William J. Robinson said that caviar is the treatment of choice in cases of nutritionally reversible impotency.

When wooden kitchen matches were used in Europe and America, the main ingredient in their manufacture was phosphorus. Men working in the match-making plant suffered from priapism, that is a painful and prolonged erection of the male genitalia.

However, phosphorus, as it is obtained from the earth, is a poison. Only when it is processed by an organism (in this case, the sturgeon) can it serve the function desired by the reader.

To set the stage for a sweet seduction,

you can plan an entire meal from appetizer to dessert using the ingredients given in this chapter. (Remember the notoriously lusty eating scene in the movie *Tom Jones*?) Don't forget the wine, candlelight, and a little chocolate couldn't hurt either. And remember, if you can't stand the heat, why not get out of the kitchen — and head for the Jacuzzi?

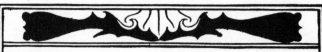

HOPSCOTCHING THE WORLD OF HERBS

Love is an irresistible desire to be irresistibly
desired.   *Robert Frost 1874–1963*

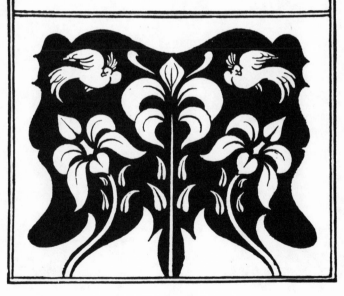

HERE'S an eye-opening introduction to a vast variety of herbs from all corners of the earth, all gathered today and in ages past with the aim of putting a little more "whoop" into makin' whoopee.

MOHO-MOHO / *Piper angustifolium*

This pepper tree grows to the height of 10 feet and is called moho-moho by the natives of Peru. They pick the leaves during the growing season and dry the leaves in the sun. Then, when sexual desire is flagging, they put a tablespoon of the dried leaves into a cup of water and let it boil for one minute. Then the cup is taken away from the heat and allowed to steep for one-half to one hour. Then it is strained, sweetened with honey and imbibed.

It owes its power to an aromatic oil and a substance called matacine.

It is obtainable in Ecuador and many other parts of Latin America under a variety of names.

Chelone glabra

This herb has a bittersweet taste, particularly the leaves which are used for their stimulating powers. Brew it into a weak tea or it will be too bitter.

MYRTLE / *Myrica cerifera*

This is a species of myrtle growing in many parts of the United States. It grows deep green leaves and bears waxy berries.

The bark of the roots is best used for passionate purposes. It should be collected in the spring because that's when most of the sap is collected in them.

A tea prepared from this plant causes "the juices to flow."

COTTON ROOT / *Gossypium herbaceum*

The inner bark contains an acid resin which turns red when exposed to the air. It is supposed to be a sexual stimulant possibly because it looks like blood.

The usual recipe calls for placing the bark in a quart of water and boiling it down to a pint. Then, a tablespoon is to be taken at bedtime.

Although this is supposed to be useful to both sexes, it seems to be more useful to the female of the species.

ACACIA / *Acacia arabica*

This is one of the early sexual supportives. The acacia gum is mixed with a little butter, honey, and spices and chewed well to mix with saliva.

Its mineral content makes it valuable.

GALANGAL / *Alpinia galanga*

This is an aromatic root now found in Southeast Asia that tastes like ginger but is warming to the genitals. For this reason, it has been used as a sexual stimulant. In the Middle Ages, lovers used this plant in cooking as we use ginger today. Try chicken, shrimp or rice galangal.

Carduus acaulis

The root is used because of its pleasant taste. It inflames the animal spirit and restores strength too.

Cymbopogon schoenanthus

Although used mostly as a perfume constituent, the fleshy part of the root is eaten as a sexual stimulant for both men and women.

Cyperus esulentus

The tuber is peeled, sliced, and boiled in some kind of soup for its aphrodisiac effect. If you prefer, you can chew on the tuber after having buttered it and flavored it with pepper.

GOAT'S RUE / Galega officinalis

One of the few sexual stimulants recommended especially for women.

Garcinia

In West Tropical Africa, the roots of this shrub are steeped in wine and taken to stimulate lust.

Hydrocotvie asiatica

This Indian and Chinese herb is used for virility and is available in most health food stores.

HONEYSUCKLE / Lonicera japonica

The flowers, vines and leaves are said to increase vitality.

CHINESE TEA TREE / Lycium chinense

The root acts on the sexual organs. Take as a decoction, once a day.

BUTTER TREE / Madhuca butyracea

In India, a mixture of one ounce of the flowers mixed with eight ounces of milk is considered to be a cure for impotence.

HORSERADISH TREE / Moringa oleifera

Throughout the West Indies the flowers of this tree are boiled with milk to cure general debility and impotence.

MAI-TUNG / *Ophiopogon japonicus*

The tubers of this plant can be candied and eaten as an aphrodisiac.

FLEECEFLOWER ROOT
Polygonum multiflorum

This root plant nourishes the essential organs of the body and improves the oxygen-carrying capacity of the blood. The starch is used by the body as a carbohydrate source of energy while the active ingredient called chrysophanol improves sexual performance.

The tubers are dried and powdered, then one teaspoon is mixed with a large glass of boiling water and left to steep for 20 minutes. Afterward, the tea is sipped.

Other methods include breaking pieces of the root into small chunks and soaking them in vodka for 10 days. Then strain the alcoholic beverage and take one tablespoon three times a day.

Do not expect results to come in a flash. Like most tonic herbs, effects come on slowly after a couple of weeks.

The Chinese use the word tonic to de-

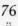

scribe the beneficial effects of certain herbs. Tonic and aphrodisiac are interchangeable in most cases.

FO-TI-TIENG

The greatest advocate — and advertisement — of this herb, Li Ch'ung-yun, is said to have lived for 256 years . . . and was still fertile to the end of his days.

He had 24 wives, loads of hair on his head, his own teeth and an erectile potential second to no man.

His advice to people was to "sit like a tortoise, walk like a pigeon, and sleep like a dog. Fast at regular intervals and except for ginseng, only eat vegetables that grow in the sunlight and nothing else."

He claimed that some of his vitality came from the herb *hydrocotyle asiatica* which he took daily as well as from fo-ti-tieng.

Fresh leaves are better than dried but unless you live in China, India or Hawaii, you'll have to settle for the dried leaves.

One teaspoon of the herb's leaves, brewed into a tea, promotes digestion, vitality and strength. Two teaspoons to a cup will gradually boost your sexual vitality.

Chinese Tonic Herbs

Every cosmopolitan city has its Chinatown. Chinese herbalists are among the most knowledgeable in the world but you should know a little about the herbs used as amorous tonics even though you may want to ask for advice. In brief, they are:

TANG KUEI / *Radix angelicae sinensis*

Highly praised and used in the Orient.
Although good for both men and women, it's thought to be the ultimate woman's tonic.

CHINESE LICORICE ROOT
Glycyrrhizae uralensis

Excellent tonic and longevity herb for men and women. May be chewed raw or cooked and made into a tea.

HO SHOU WU / *Polygonum multiflorum*

Used by millions regularly. It has a strong reputation as a youth preserver, rejuvenator and sexual tonic.

It may be eaten raw or taken as sugar-coated pills.

SCHIZANDRA FRUCTUS
Schizandra chinensis

A youth preserver, beautifier and powerful sexual tonic.

Soak in pure water for several hours before using. Take a handful of the berries and place them in a pot of water for two hours. Then throw out the water and rinse the berries. Add three cups of fresh water plus a slice of licorice root. Add an equal amount of lycii berries. Simmer for 15 minutes.

Drink a cup of tea daily for three months to build your sexual energy.

LYCII FRUCTUS / *Lycium chinensis*

Lycii berries should be vibrant red in color. If they're brown-red they have been standing too long to do you any good. If they're dry and crunchy, they're too old.

Make a brew of lycii and schizandra in equal parts for one of China's best tonics.

ASTRAGALI RADIX
Astragalus membranaceus

For your essential energy and essentially for the younger person who finds that once is enough. It can be combined with ginseng for an extra boost.

To build strength and muscle along with sexual drive, combine with codonopsitis, atractylus and licorice root.

CODONOPSITIS RADIX / *Codonopsitis*

This is a general tonic used to restore body vigor. Its activity is similar to ginseng. It is part of a powerful tonic known as Dragon Herbal. To make it mix equal parts of codonopsitis, poria cocus, atractylus, and honey-fried licorice.

The combination is one of the best energy tonics ever developed and is also very tasty.

ATRACTYLUS / *Atractylodis ovata*

For energy, sexual stimulation and digestion.

SUK GOK / *Dendrobium hancockii*

The stems of this Chinese orchid are said to be stimulating and help replace lost energy. Rinse the herb then mix with licorice root. Simmer for about 20 minutes or until the tea is rich and good tasting.

PORIA / *Poria cocos*

This is not truly an herbal since it is a solid, pulpy fungus which grows on the roots of the fir tree. However, it restores and refreshes the body and the mind. Poria helps regulate the fluids of the genito-urinary system thereby contributing to reproductive health and lovemaking.

TU-CHUNG / *Eucommia ulmoides*

This dried bark is very difficult to obtain because it's being studied by a number of American drug companies for its ability to lower blood pressure. Its active ingredient, with no discovered side effects, is an improvement over reserpine.

Besides its ability to regulate blood pressure, this herb is very popular as a sexual tonic.

SHAN CHU-YU / *Cornus officinalis*

Cornus is a tonic which acts upon the genito-urinary system. This herb controls sperm ejaculation and strengthens the lower body.

Dioscoria Batatas

This herb contains certain steroid precursors and is useful when the body has less hormone activity than is desired.

Ligusticum lucidum

This herb improved circulation, particularly to the genito-urinary tract, thereby improving circulation to the male organ of copulation.

Ligusticum also improves the functioning of the nervous system. Both qualities are important to an improved sex life.

TREE PEONY / *Paeonia suffruticosa*

This herb is from the bark of the tree and is beneficial mostly to the female, particularly if she wishes to conceive.

GOTU-KOLA / *Centella asiatica*

The Chinese say that two leaves of the plant *Centella asiatica* keep old age away and millions of Chinese make a practice of enjoying this herb every day of their lives.

A daily cup of tea made with a teaspoon or two of the leaves is an excellent tonic to the brain and the body. It stimulates the hormonal system, helps digestion, improves resistance to disease and, if sexual energy is on the wane, it boosts vitality and increases enjoyment.

What more can you ask from a couple of of leaves?

Praxinus excelsior

The leaves of this tree mixed in wine and flavored with powdered nutmeg have the reputation of "stirring up lust for the opposite sex."

Orobanche ammophyla

Wild stallions in the heat of amorous occupation dropped their seed on the ground and from the semen sprang this plant.

Perhaps it didn't really happen this way, but those who eat the plant's root swear by its ability to strengthen them for love and to cure those afflicted by an inability to consummate the conjugal act.

ORIENTAL CASHEW TREE
Semecarpus anacardium

This plant has tasty seeds and the nuts contain sustaining nutrients which are said to help maintain reproductive power into the 90s.

CHINESE RASPBERRY

In the central and western provinces of China there grow special raspberries which are picked and dried. The fresh fruit benefits the lungs and circulation while the dried fruit is said to have aphrodisiac abilities.

Withania somnifera

A pinch of the powdered root mixed with milk and honey is recommended for impotence. This plant contains an alkaloid called

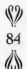

somniferine and should be used with care. It can be taken as a tea by boiling some of the powdered root in water for 10 minutes. Then strain and sweeten with some honey. Sip the tea before meals twice a day.

❧ Beyond the Orient ❧

PERIWINKLE / *Vinca minor*

A few years ago, acting on legends derived from Gypsy folklore that this plant was effective against the ravages of diabetes, the medical community began to investigate its active ingredients. Although it was not found to be effective against diabetes, an alkaloid was uncovered that has shown great promise against a host of diseases including leukemia and certain types of viral infections.

A brew of periwinkle was used in Hungary as a marital aid for the overtired.

IGNATIUS BEAN / *Strychnos ignatii*

Danger and sex make a great combination. People have risked death by eating the flesh of the fugu (blow fish) in Japan on the off chance that it can excite their flagging sexual interest. Some achieve their goal while others are carried out of the restaurant to the grave.

So it is with the ignatius bean which contains strychnine. Strychnine is a violent poison which, in tiny doses, is also a nerve and muscle tonic. In the smallest of doses it's capable of restoring natural power and energy . . . in larger doses, goodbye!

Tacca involucrata

Only the royal family of some African tribes was allowed the privilege of chomping on the tuber of this plant because it not only revived lost lust, but allegedly provided only male children as a result of that lust.

That's a lot to ask of a plant.

Securinega virosa

Before Rhodesia became Zimbabwe, natives cultivated this plant for its aphrodisiac qualities. Today, its citizens still claim
that the root, brewed into a strong tea, has
the ability to excite the senses—especially
among the older generation. Although there
has been no scientific investigation into
the active ingredients, the custom still pre-
vails and appears to have some validity.

Saussurea lappa

The ancient Malays had no laboratories to
test the active ingredients found in the
many plant species in Malaya, now Malaysia. Their only laboratories were their
bodies; the only proof was in sustained
erections. Plant after plant was given the
acid test. If it worked, the witch doctor
had another tool, so to speak, in his
arsenal.

Saussurea contains an essential oil which,
when excreted through the penis along with
the urine, is an irritant. Apparently the
irritation is accompanied by an erection.
So, no matter how it is arrived at, the

witch doctor collects his substantial fee for obtaining the desired result.

Iodoicea sechellarum

Palm trees bear coconuts. This exceptionally tall palm tree bears exceptionally heavy nuts, some weighing as much as 50 pounds, taking up to 10 years to ripen. Walking under such a palm tree is a hazard, for when the nuts fall they hit with a force that splits the earth and they bury themselves.

Later a long shoot grows from the nut in order to begin a new tree. The fruit, which has a rather so-so flavor, is said to be an aphrodisiac and was once favored as a pre-fling treat in the harems of India.

SALEP / *Sahlab*

This herb is venerated in Turkey for its restorative powers which reportedly give males the ability to satisfy many women at one laying.

The roots, when boiled in water, form a mucilaginous mass like a thickened jelly. This jelly is esteemed also in India where it is called one of the finest tonic aphrodisiacs for people who have lost their sexual powers.

A combination of salep, basil leaves and cardamom powder in goat's milk is said to have been so powerful, a handful of noodles placed in the broth stood erect for 20 minutes before finally relaxing.

Of course this is a folktale, illustrating the power that legend confers on a mixture that has been reported effective for so many cases.

Women who have lost interest in sex should prepare this combination and sip it three times a day.

Linum usitatissimum

The use of this herb requires some preparation and a good cook since it must be mixed with honey and red pepper and turned into a muffin.

Finally, it doesn't appear to be worth the effort since there are so many other recommended herbs and a muffin with pepper isn't very appetizing.

Eryngium comosum

This herb can be used in a number of ways to arouse the reluctant male organ. Juice can be squeezed from the root, mixed with butter and honey and taken by the tablespoonful. Or you can boil a piece of the root in water for 10 minutes and make into a tea. The tea may be sweetened with honey unless you like the bitter taste.

Since this herb is also a diuretic, be prepared for many trips to the john in between making merry with Mary.

Myrtus communis

One of the selected plants for the goddess Venus and venerated as a love tonic since ancient times.

The leaves are macerated with any sweet alcoholic beverage and sipped before an amorous adventure. It is said to be able to add fire where only coals are to be found and to cause blazing passion where fire is found.

Nandina domestica

Another Chinese herb with a good reputation. This one is an evergreen with classical red berries which follow large, showy white flowers. It is both a medicinal shrub and a foliage shrub.

The leaves and branches are made into a tea by infusion in boiling water to drive away that tired feeling at the end of the day. That should be enough to recommend its use. But it is also good when you have a cold. And, to complete the menu, the seeds, macerated in a warm brandy, strengthen virility.

If you live in a temperate climate you can plant this shrub and enjoy its luxuriant foliage at the same time that you take advantage of its strengthening potential.

Averrhoa carambola

This herb appears to have multiple uses since the powdered seeds, made into a tea, act as a sexual stimulant but the same seeds in larger doses can be an abortofacient.

Its third use is as an intoxicant, although

that may be because it's dissolved in alcohol instead of water.

Tinospora cordifolia

According to India's Ayurvedic medicine, this creeper plant is one of the most useful to excite the libido. The plant is most effective when used in its fresh state. The leaves and bark make a stimulant tea while the roots offer a starch substance which can be made into cake-like buns which are eaten as a prelude to passion.

Tribulus terrestris

The whole plant is useful to establish connubial bliss. The fruit, the roots and the leaves are mixed together in a pot with sufficient water and boiled for seven minutes. The mixture is then strained and set aside to cool. The resulting tea is taken in large glasses twice a day.

Another method is to use the plant as a vegetable to be eaten with boiled rice. Some randy wives, desiring to increase their husbands' conjugal visits, use the plant for food without telling their spouse. It's a sneaky but very clever way to attain their end without appearing to be wanton.

Sphaeranthus hirtus

This remedy takes a while to prepare.

Take the fresh root of the plant and steep it in tepid water overnight. Then place the root in oil and heat the oil until the last drop of moisture is expelled. Slice the root into tiny pieces and take one tiny piece first thing in the morning for 30 days, meanwhile abstaining from any sexual contact.

At the end of the month, the desire to copulate should be sufficiently stimulated.

(Why not just go to jail for 30 days?)

Veronica officinalis

When tea leaves were in short supply in Germany, the leaves of this plant were steeped in hot water and used as a substitute.

After drinking the tea, some people were provoked to charge into the bedroom. This led to the belief that the tea has definite stimulating action. Modern books list this plant as a blood purifier but the proof is in the drinking.

PLANTAIN / *Plantago major*

Common plantago is sometimes recommended to increase virility perhaps because of the fruit's suggestive shape.

For an infusion, steep one teaspoon fresh or dried leaves in half a cup of water. Take one cup a day, a mouthful at a time.

Or drink two to three cups of the juice a day.

PRIDE OF CHINA *or* CHINABERRY
Melia azedarach

The tree exudes a gum which has been considered to be an aphrodisiac. But beware: Chinaberries are poisonous.

QUEEN OF THE MEADOW *or* MARSH MILKWEED
Eupatorium purpureum

American Indian tribes used this plant when they wanted to rock their tee-pees.

To make an infusion, steep one ounce of the root in one pint of water for 30 minutes. Take one ounce three times a day. Or use as a tincture. Take eight to 15 drops daily as needed.

MATICO / *Piper angustifolium*

This herb is a favorite aphrodisiac among Peruvians.

Use one teaspoon of the leaves to one cup of water to make an infusion. Take one to two cups a day.

FENUGREEK / *Trigonella foenumgraecum*

This herb has been considered an aphrodisiac since ancient times.

Fenugreek Decoction

Use two teaspoons of seeds with one cup of cold water; let stand for five hours.
Then boil for just one minute.
Take two to three cups daily.
The decoction's taste is improved by adding some peppermint essence or honey.

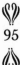

WORMWOOD / *Artemisia absinthium*

This is the active ingredient in the French drink called absinthe. The oil of wormwood is considered to be both aphrodisiac and poisonous. The flowering tops are used to make a tea which is considered to be almost as effective and much less liable to be poisonous, providing only a weak tea is prepared and ingested.

Durio zibethinus

In Indonesia, Sumatra, the Celebes, the Moluccas, Borneo and its environs, there grows a spiny fruit which is considered by many to be one of the strongest aphrodisiacs in the world.

Providing you can beat the natives to it, and you can muster enough courage to eat it once you've smelled it.

Some people have said the odor resembles that of the smelliest cheese in the world, gorgonzola, at its ripest.

Or smelly socks, cheese and onions.

Or custard that has travelled the sewers of France.

But all of them agree that the flavor is out of this world.

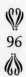

If you can fight off the natives and the animals, which also want to partake of its pulp, you may find an aphrodisiac which can raise the dead.

Eugenia crenulata

The leaves of this shrub are steeped in rum by the poorer people who can't afford a trip to the witch doctor for an expensive sexual stimulant. It's popular especially in Haiti.

Also, after drinking the rum, a small bundle of leaves is tied together in the form of a charm or wanga. Between the charm and the drink, amorous relations are almost ensured.

Grewua umbellata

All countries have their popular plant that helps restore virility and Thailand is no different. Thais use all parts of this low-growing shrub, mixing leaves or bark with the native sour drink.

KAVA-KAVA / *Piper methysticum*

In the South Pacific are a string of islands that seem to exude sexuality. Reinforced by motion pictures from Hollywood in the forties, they appeared to be hotbeds of romantic tussles.

If that was and is the true picture, perhaps it is helped by a potion made from the root of the kava-kava plant.

Piper methysticum grows best near sea level in areas like Samoa, Tahiti and Fiji. The stimulating ingredients are in the roots which, with sufficient sunlight and three to four years' growth, can be up to five inches thick.

Although rare, plants that have seen 20 or more island summers can have heavy, knotted roots that can weigh up to 100 pounds. These are sought after as the best aphrodisiac possible. When harvested, the roots are then scraped and cut into tiny pieces which are then either pounded into pulp or chewed until mushy.

We are more civilized and have a blender to work with. The idea of chewing roots and spitting the results into a common pot for common usage is best suited to the Tonga tribe. So here's a recipe for:

**Kava-kava
"Tonight's the Night" Fizz**

Put one ounce of chopped or ground root
in a blender and add:
two tablespoons of a bland vegetable oil
one tablespoon lecithin flakes
one-half cup skim milk
one-half cup water
some chopped ice
Blend thoroughly and strain.
This recipe makes about two cups of joy.

This mixture evokes a climate of warmth and is gently stimulating to the genital area. Don't drink your stimulating portion more than an hour before your proposed encounter because in two hours you'll be fast asleep and counting dream girls, not live ones.

Kava-kava's activity is attributed to a collection of alpha pyrones. Although insoluble in water, the beating action of the blender distributes them throughout the mixture. The milky appearance of the mixture tells you your love potion is ready to drink.

If you have good teeth and prefer to prepare it the way they do in the islands . . . good luck!

MUSK SEEDS / *Hibiscus moschatus*

This seed grows in a five-cornered pyramid capsule and looks like a striped snail shell. It's called musk seed because it smells and tastes like musk, so appealing that the seeds are sometimes chewed to sweeten the breath.

It's considered to be an aphrodisiac by the Arabs and can be ground and brewed with water or milk.

GARDEN HELIOTROPE
Valeriana officinalis

A mildly potent aphrodisiac. Take one-half ounce of the root and boil it in a covered pot for five or six minutes, then strain.

What's the problem?

The taste is passable but the stench is enough to make strong men weep and women flee.

Heliotrope contains chatinine (not bad), valerine (tolerable) and valeric acid (resembles old socks worn for 30 days by each member of the Dallas Cowboys in turn without washing).

If there ever was an aphrodisiac that was an anaphrodisiac . . . this is it.

Maybe old timers believed it had to be "bad" to do some "good."

CEREUS CACTUS
Selenicereus grandiflorus

The fleshy cactus does have grand flowers when it blooms. The sight is a pleasure to behold: Giant blossoms up to a foot or more across with scintillating aroma that is reminiscent of vanilla.

They open at night, yielding their fragrance to the moon. Six hours later they fold their blossoms and dry.

These cactus flowers and their stems are useful when coital ability has been temporarily lost due to overactivity or exhaustion (happy thought).

Five drops of the fresh juice is said to revive a flaccid member . . . 10 drops will revive a dead member.

Or, chew on a bit of the stem.

Or, mix some of the flowers and stem

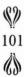

with some vodka and have a slug or two.

But—take too much and risk delirium. Always start at the lowest dose.

COCKSCOMB
Celosia argentea

A decoction of the seeds is used as an aphrodisiac in the Philippines.

VELVET LEAF
Chasmanthera owariensis

African women who suspect their spouse's affections are waning use this root.

PEGA PALO
Rhynchosia phaseolodes

In the Dominican Republic, lazy would-be lovers are to steep one inch of the vine in a bottle of rum for one week. Then sip one jiggerful three times a day.

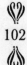

Carduus acaulis

The young leaves are eaten in Japan as a stimulant.

Costus speciosus

The powdered herb is taken internally in the Malay Islands as an aphrodisiac.

SENSITIVE PLANT / Mimosa pudica

This plant is found in many American homes because of its curious habit of responding to the touch. We call it sensitive or touch-me-not plant. The tribes of the Amazon jungle also cultivate the sensitive plant but for other reasons. The roots give off a juice that is applied to the feet or genitals to provide more orgasms and greater stamina.

The mimosa plant contains tryptamines and the Peruvians make a tea from the leaves for the same purpose, but the plant grows in two forms: the male form excites and the female form relaxes.

The difficulty for us is in telling the difference. Plants have no trouble telling which is which, but it would be a shame to make a tea of one when you really need the other.

The prize for unlikely sources of aphrodisiacs seems to go to our Native Americans, the Apaches, who favored cow dung for their love magic. Strangely enough, a company in the West is selling purified cow dung in 10-pound sacks. The odor is quite pleasant and surprisingly stimulating, like a musky perfume. So maybe the Apaches had something after all.

DODDER / *Cuscuta*

The seeds of all species of this parasitic plant have long been used in China as a sexual stimulant.

CEYLON SAGO / *Cycas circinalis*

When dried, the scales of this plant can be intoxicant and aphrodisiac.

DURIAN / *Durio zibethinus*

The spiny fruit of the durio tree has been used as an aphrodisiac in Indonesia, Su-

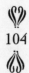

matra, the Moluccas, the Celebes and in Borneo.

Americans who have tried the fruit say two things: The fruit smells like rotting flesh, but has a most delicious taste.

BARRENWORT / *Epimedium sagittatum*

The aphrodisiac qualities of this plant were discovered by startled onlookers who were watching goats in action after they had eaten the leaves. The Chinese use the roots and the leaves.

GARDEN ROCKET / *Eruca sativa*

Once used as a stimulant tonic only, it was prescribed for monks who suffered from fatigue. After a daily dose of the infusion the monks were found to be trangressing their vows.

WATER ERYNGO / *Eryngium aquaticum*

Prescribed for sexual exhaustion and loss of erectile power.

LOVAGE / *Levisticum officinale*

As an infusion, use one teaspoon of the fresh or dried root to one cup of water. Take one cup daily.

Bath Decoction

Boil two ounces of the root
in five quarts of water
for use in a bath.

Not for pregnant women or those with kidney problems.

INDIAN MALLOW / *Abutilon indicum*

Use the leaves to make a decoction.

BEAD TREE *or* RED SANDALWOOD
Adenanthera pavonina

Use a decoction of the leaves or the bark.

ARABIAN MANNA / *Alhagi maurorum*

Sweet exudation found on the leaves has been used as a sexual stimulant.

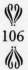

PRINCE'S-FEATHERS
Amaranthus hybridus

Use the leaves, roots or seeds to make a decoction.

HOPS / *Humulus lupulus*

This is the hops which is added to beer during the brewing process to produce the beer flavor and some of its intoxicating power which is so popular among fraternity men.

Beer is not known for its ability to enhance the lovemaking ability of its drinkers. In fact, it's said to lower the ability to satisfy the beer drinker's partner even if the beer drinker makes it into the bedroom. But in this case, the part is greater than the whole.

The hop plant is a relative of cannabis (marijuana) and, if rolled into a cigarette and smoked, will produce a mild high accompanied by a sense of serenity.

For more lecherous purposes follow the following procedure:

107

> ### Hops Potion
> Take one ounce of hops.
> Let steep in a pint of tepid water for
> 70 minutes.
> Strain.
> Take a teaspoonful before sex.

A little will help, but a tablespoonful will put a lid on any lovemaking. If you can't sleep, however, a tablespoonful at bedtime will have you snoring in minutes.

As usual, avoid overdosing. More is not better and can lead to dizziness and some signs of jaundice. Hops contains as its active ingredient the substance called lupuline, a yellow resin that is a close relative to THC. This accounts for its ability to present everything in a better light and let the libido out of the closet.

CARLINE THISTLE / *Carlina acaulis*

This plant has been prescribed in the past as a cure for impotence.

For an infusion, take six teaspoons of the

rootstock to one cup of water. Drink one or two cups daily.

Thistle Decoction

Use one teaspoon rootstock to
one-half cup of water.
Boil briefly. Cool.
Take one to two cups a day,
one mouthful at a time.

Or take 10 drops on a sugar cube or in water three times a day as a tincture. To use the powdered form, put one-quarter to one-half teaspoon in water two to three times a day.

SUNDEW / *Drosera rotundifolia*

This insectivorous plant is an aphrodisiac according to some European traditions. The fresh juice is taken internally.

But sundew contains irritating substances and should only be used in tiny amounts.

EUROPEAN VERVAIN / *Verbena officinalis*

This perennial has been used to secure the favor of the ladies for centuries.

Cold Extract

Soak one tablespoon of the plant
in one cup of water for eight to 10 hours.
Take one cup a day

Tincture

Take 10 to 20 drops in water
two to three times a day.
Or take one-quarter teaspoon of the
powdered plant
two to three times a day.

IBOGA / *Tabernanthe iboga*

Remember the song, "I could have danced all night"? It could have originated in Africa among the people who use this herb as a stimulating aphrodisiac. Africans who drink iboga in all-night ceremonies that include vigorous dancing and even more vigorous sex may stay up the next day and night until the stimulation wears off.

Eventually they fall into a deep, satiated sleep which can last for 18 hours.

Ibogaine is the active ingredient of this tropical shrub that is found in the Congo and also Gabon. It's been used for hundreds of years and its action is similar to that of yohimbine. Ibogaine is an indole alkaloid and is illegal in the United States.

As is true for many herbals, the activity depends on the dose. A small amount, less than one gram of the root or bark, acts as an aphrodisiac. Users claim it is a cure for impotence.

Users also claim that the iboga can grant enough sexual strength to engage in non-stop sexual activity for up to 16 hours!

Now for the bad news: An overdose can bring on convulsions, paralysis, or even death from respiratory failure.

KAT *or* KHAT / *Catha edulis*

What amphetamine is to speed freaks, the buds, leaves and stems of this large shrub (a relative of the burning bush family) is to natives of Ethiopia and surrounding areas. Khat is a central nervous system stimulant, a bit on the mild side probably due to the presence of a lot of vitamin C, which minimizes the effects of cathine, cathidine and cathinine.

The word is still out on whether or not this herb is a true aphrodisiac. Some people say yes and others say no. Some report happy experiences while others say it works against good sex. Aborigines chewed the bitter leaves for stimulation.

So, if you're in Ethiopia and someone puts the Khat out, better pass.

SPANISH PELLITORY
Anacyclus pyrethrum or Anthemis pyrethrum

Both names are given to prevent confusion with other herbs.

The herb we're investigating is Spanish pellitory and it has a history that goes back to the ancient Romans. Ovid mentions Spanish pellitory with caution, equating it with the very dangerous Spanish fly. Other sources have it as one of the best herbals to restore one's ability "to attack the sacred mount" more quickly than if you depend on nature alone. When in Rome, you'll not be able to try this remedy because it's not to be found. However, when in India . . .

COLA NUT / *Cola nitida*

This herbal was the cola of Coca-Cola, but is no longer an ingredient in that or any other American drink. However, it's still used as a beverage in Brazil and in Jamaica it's used as a sexual stimulant.

That's not its only use. It's a condiment (the seeds are powdered and sprinkled on food), it's a digestive in the West Indies, and is used to heal small cuts in Brazil.

Cola or kola contains *a lot* of caffeine, theobromine, and kolanin. The kolanin is a source of energy, helping to burn fats and carbohydrates in the body.

One teaspoon of the powder can be added to a strong cup of coffee for all the energy you need for a full night of love. So don't plan on a "quickie" and a snooze. Cola is a strong stimulant.

Stimulants work by causing nerve fibers to release noradrenaline and other stimulating neurotransmitters. Although different stimulants bring about this release in different ways, the end result is the same: the release of more stimulating neurotransmitters. It's the body's energy going to work in the nervous system.

The release of noradrenaline causes predictable changes in the mind and the body. You'll feel wakeful, alert, and often very happy. There will be a rush of excitement, a sense of increased mental and physical energy.

How you use that energy and increased awareness is up to you.

CALEA / *Calea zacatechichi*

The Chontal Indians of Oaxaca are not slouches when it comes to stimulation. They use a shrub from the sunflower family which grows from Costa Rica to Central Mexico for a flagging libido as well as a mild hallucinogen.

Try a teaspoonful of the leaves in a pint of water, boil for five minutes, then strain and sip a little.

POTENTWOOD *or* MUIRIA PUAMA
Lyriosma ovata

This may be one of the more tested of the herbal products, since it appears in the Brazilian pharmacopoeia as a possible remedy for impotence and has been used for centuries along the Amazon.

The parts used are the inner bark and wood of the tree commonly called Muiria puama but botanically known as *Lyriosma ovata*.

A strong decoction is made from the bark and wood. This is rubbed on the genitals to act as a central nervous stimulant.

The result of this rubbing may depend on who is doing the rubbing. If another party, perhaps the decoction is not needed after all.

A fluid extract is also made from the bark and the wood and given in daily doses of about 10 drops.

There is a product on the market in Germany composed of potentwood, testicular tissue, anterior pituitary extract, lecithin, cola extract, yohimbine hydrochloride, calcium lactate and strychnine. It's sold in Latin America as a sex aid.

Outside of the fact that the active ingredient is a resin, little is scientifically known about the contents except that its power is extractable with alcohol. An ounce of the herb can be placed in a jar with a couple of cups of vodka and left there for about two weeks. Shake daily and, when done, have a shot before making love.

Or, take two tablespoonsful of the powdered wood and boil it in water for 15 minutes. A shot of this mixture taken half an hour before lovemaking can produce the earth-shaking results you are looking for.

JIMSONWEED / *Datura stramonium*

Do not use without medical supervision. In South America, jimsonweed is said to have aphrodisiac powers, but this plant is poisonous.

Virola calophylla

Mother Nature has been kind in providing a wide assortment of plant products for man's use. Wide experimentation by indigenous peoples has resulted in many different substances from the leaves, bark, roots and seeds. However, some trees also give off resins which have been experimented with. Epena, from the *Virola calophylla*, is one such resin.

Natives of the Amazon scrape a red resin

from the tree after first ceremoniously removing some of the bark. (The tree is a
member of the nutmeg family which is
interesting because nutmeg does have some
amorous ability in itself.)

After the resin has been thoroughly dried,
which takes a few days, it is pounded into
a fine powder and then mixed with ashes
from a wood fire. The result is much like
the snuff available in tobacco stores.

However, it is a fast-acting stimulant
which has nothing to do with tobacco. The
user is intoxicated with beauty and a variety of sensations. Pleasure is heightened
and even the slightest touch can inspire a
rapturous interval.

Euphoria can last after the sex act is
completed, but the resinous snuff is not
without its unpleasant effects.

Because it's snorted, it severely irritates
the sensitive mucous membrane, causing
uncontrollable sneezing. (It's one thing to
sneeze but sneezing during other spasms
may complicate the experience and drive
your partner away.)

Since this method of obtaining a pleasure trip has been shown to be possibly
unpleasant in the beginning, some users

have chosen another route to instill pleasure. Some of the snuff is dissolved in water and administered anally thereby circumventing the nasal passages.

This is a potent MAO inhibitor.

DITA / *Alstonia scholaris*

Like the tree which yields yohimbine, the bark of this tall (70 feet or higher) tree has been used for ages. From the Philippines to India, decoctions of the bark have been used to treat women afflicted with painful menstrual cramps. But the tree, being impartial, also is an aid to men suffering from the inability to maintain an erection and from premature ejaculation. In the latter case it's the seeds which are used.

The active ingredient in the seeds is called chlorogenine and can be extracted by crushing and then soaking the seeds in water for 24 hours. The strained liquid is taken a tablespoon at a time (no more than three tablespoons) before sex.

Use no more than one gram of the crushed seed when preparing your potion.

SEA HOLLY / *Eryngium maritimum*

Candied sea holly roots were used in England about the time of Shakespeare to help renew the amorous ability of mature males. Its ability to act as a diuretic led to its more fanciful use as an aphrodisiac, since the roots do have a shape that resembles an erect penis.

Use two little rootlets and boil them for five minutes in water. Or soak them in wine for 12 hours, then strain and drink the wine.

 Hallucinogenic Aphrodisiacs

During the era of herbs, particularly the 16th and 17th centuries, doctors and botanists examined many types of plants, searching for "magic potions." The age of exploration took them into the mountains and the jungles where they uncovered hundreds of exotic "mental" aphrodisiacs. The process of discovery continued into present times, uncovering native herbals with the alleged power to increase sexual ability in the physical sense as well as blowing the mind.

This section deals with the ethnopharmacology of obscure aphrodisiacs used by many uncivilized cultures. However, in many cases the cure might have been worse than the disease, because some of these remedies are poisonous.

Amanita Muscaria or Amanita Pantherina

These are part of a family of wild mushrooms; some are edible and some are deadly.

In Siberia, where not many herbs can grow, primitive tribes of long ago discovered the intoxicant qualities hidden in the highly toxic amanita or fly agaric mushroom.

The mushroom cap can be dried and smoked; the mushroom can be eaten fresh, cooked or dried; it can be made into a tea. Each preparation produces a different result.

Moderate doses usually cause a type of dreamy intoxication with everything beautiful and easy.

But high doses are dangerous, even deadly, so this is not a recommended aphrodisiac.

The chemicals in the mushroom have

been isolated in the laboratory and identified as ibotenic acid and muscimol, substances that resemble GABA (gamma
aminobutyric acid), one of the brain's
own neurotransmitters. It's strange to
think that nature has duplicated our brain
chemicals in a mushroom, but that's
not the strangest part of the fly agaric
culture.

Among the Koryak people of Siberia,
urine-drinking parties are held on their
festive occasions. Considering the fact that
mushrooms are hard to find in such a cold
climate, the idea of recycling their aphrodisiacal abilities until exhausted may not
be so repugnant.

Here's how it goes:

They collect a bunch of mushrooms, pour
water on them and then boil them until
the chief thinks all of the power has passed
into the water. Then the chief and the
most important people at the party drink
the intoxicating liquid.

After a time they have to urinate. This
urine is collected in a "sacred" bowl and
passed out to the next in importance . . .
and so on until everyone at the party is in
a state of intoxication.

(Can this be the origin of being "pissed off"?)

About 4,000 years ago, trade began between those Siberian tribes and the people living in the Indus Valley of neighboring India. The use of fly agaric may have then spread to India since the sacred book of India, the *Rig Veda*, contains the following quote:

Like a stag, come here to drink!
Drink Soma, as much as you like.
Pissing it out day by day, O generous one,
You have assumed your most mighty force.

For our purposes, the mushrooms' dangers far outweigh the possible pleasure to be obtained. More people die from ingestion of poisonous mushroons than benefit from them. Although the danger is much greater with *A. pantherina* than with *A. muscaria*, either one can be a killer.

Pedalium murex

India supplies another plant whose seed, fruit and leaves are commonly used as a soothing diuretic but, when prepared in a special manner, the plant has aphrodisiacal effects.

Love Tonic
Crush one part seeds and put
in 20 parts of water.
Let stand for 24 hours, then filter.
Add two ounces vodka as a preservative.
Take one teaspoonful three times a day
to stimulate the genitalia.

BETEL NUTS / *Piper betle*

Not for those who like white teeth; chewing this seed of a tropical palm blackens the teeth. So what's so attractive about a man with black teeth? Consider the stimulating properties, the mood-enhancing effect, the aphrodisiac quality of betel nuts.

When you mix betel nut with a pinch of lime and a lot of saliva, the active ingredient arecoline is released. This excites the central nervous system, increases the respiration, lifts the spirits—makes you dribble on your best shirt.

The copious flow of red juice which you spit out at frequent intervals supposedly adds to your appeal. If this is your game,

123

add a bit of nutmeg for taste and find someone who doesn't mind a dribbler.

Lest you think we're giving betel nut chewing a bad name, millions of Asians use it daily and thoroughly enjoy it as much as we enjoy our daily coffee. The workers who harvest the nuts take "sex breaks" the way we take coffee breaks, so let's not knock the cola of another society . . . maybe black teeth have their benefits after all.

SWEET FLAG, SWEET SEDGE, RAT ROOT
Calamus or Acorus calamus

This is a 2,000-year-old herb that has been used in China and in the Ayurvedic system of medicine for diseases of the lungs such as bronchitis and asthma. But there are other uses, discovered by languishing lovers desiring more and better sex.

Calamus contains an essential oil which is mainly composed of two psychoactive substances called asarone and beta-asarone. Small amounts of the root *and small amounts only*, act as stimulant to the nervous system and the libido.

The Cree Indians in Alberta chew tiny

portions of the root regularly as an anti-fatigue medicine, but large amounts can act as a mind-altering substance. No sense taking a sexual trip alone. You might not like the partner you find . . .

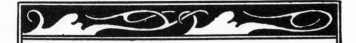

EXPOSED: SECRETS OF LEGENDARY LOVERS

All lovers swear more performance than they
are able . . .   *William Shakespeare 1564–1616*

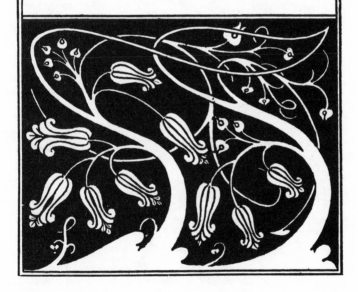

WHO HASN'T heard of Casanova, Don Juan, Cleopatra or Henry VIII? What made them live on in fact and fantasy?

Answer: Their mysterious powers of seduction and the way they reportedly satisfied themselves and their lovers . . . again and again.

How did they accomplish these amorous (and, as legend records it, often outrageous and fantastical) feats?

Answer: They knew how to use herbal and spice aphrodisiacs as part of their seductive art.

Suspend your scientific judgement and silence your inner critic for a moment to enjoy the exciting exploits of these notorious lovers. The stories that have come down to us are part fact, part fancy, and it's hard to tell at times which is which. Just savor them, and see if perhaps you can't learn just a little about pleasing your spouse or paramour from these legendary lechers.

Don Juan was a 14th-century aristocrat who was born in Seville, Spain. He had the special ability to make love to one maiden after another, competing with much

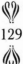

younger men and able to succeed where they had failed. Even at the advanced age of 60 to 70 he was still tops in amorous activity.

According to written reports which surfaced after his death, he credited a particular mixture with the power to restore his potency time after time. It had to be mixed fresh and taken one hour before his next encounter.

Don Juan's Secret Passion Potion

Take one-quarter teaspoon of crushed basil leaves and one cup of freshly squeezed tomato juice.
Mix furiously until the fragrance from the basil has entirely entered the juice.
Sip slowly until the potion works its way to the genital area.

Now this is the published version of Don Juan's fantastic love potion. It's possible that not all of the ingredients were revealed. The Don was a tricky fellow and was careful not to reveal the secret during his lifetime. Did he add some cinnamon, Chinese licorice or perhaps some ginseng?

Or is this the entire potion, able to do for you what it did for the Don?

Casanova was born in 1725 and died in 1798. He died in the company of three women doing what he did best to the last. Next to the bed, in a royal purple vase, was a mysterious liquid. Casanova would frequently drink of this liquid, offering wine to his guests instead.

Was this the secret to his bedroom prowess, the key to how he was able to bed more than one woman at a time?

Although analysis was not as good in the 1700s as today, some enterprising fellow made off with the vase after his death. He took it to the chemist and they believe this was the formula:

Casanova's Cocktail

one-half cup fresh grapefruit juice
one-half cup steamed apple juice
one-half teaspoonful of cinnamon powder
Mix vigorously, then sip.

Was there a secret ingredient the chemist failed to find? Or did he find it and merely give this formula to the thief? There are rumors that a chemist became the greatest lover in Italy after the death of Casanova. Could it have been the chemist who had a shot at this famous elixir of love?

First Julius fell to her charms and then it was Marc Antony's turn. What was it about Cleopatra that made men fall at her feet — then into her boudoir? Legend has it that she would prepare a potion for her lovers that promoted "unendurable pleasure, indefinitely prolonged."

However, it was not a potion for her lovers alone. She also would partake of the mixture and meet each demand with a counterdemand of her own. Although well into her fourth decade, she performed with the vigor and sexual response of an adolescent.

What was this mystical brew that made men greater lovers than they had ever been? A special maid would put together the following mixture. It had to be mixed vigorously and, after mixing, was shaken for 10 minutes by a robust Nubian slave who enjoyed the confidence of his mistress.

Nowadays we have a blender that can do the job more quickly.

Cleopatra's Elixir of Everlasting Love

In a blender place:
   one-quarter cup bananas, squashed
         thoroughly
one-quarter cup watermelon juice, no seeds
   one-half cup unripe papaya juice
   one-half teaspoonful powdered cloves
      Blend at high speed until
         thoroughly mixed.
   Sip slowly before engaging
      in a carnal cuddle.

Farfetched?

Not nutritionally speaking, since the combination of minerals, protein, vitamins in the fruit plus the natural ingredients in the cloves combine to produce a stimulant to the sex glands and hormones. Experts have told us that Cleopatra would frequently go on a 24-hour fast existing solely on this potion and no other food. Then the Queen of the Nile would reemerge from her boudoir to give and receive another 24-hour pleasure trip.

Is this the ultimate formula? Was there

another secret ingredient plucked from the gardens of the Nile and added by the maid or the slave?

Try it and see what you think.

Another queen, the dark Queen of Sheba, was able to charm King Solomon into the bed chamber and their lovemaking was so satisfying that trade treaties were made between the Hebrew nation and the land of Sheba.

It's said that a love brew prepared in secret by a special group of servants skilled in magic was the key to her stamina and the stallion-like stamina of her partners. Three times a day her servants prepared the potion for her and the king. Because it had to be prepared fresh, vegetables were gathered from the nearby fields three times a day as well.

Fortunately, one slave escaped from Sheba and founded a potion shop in what's now known as Great Britain where she achieved great success with the nobles. This is the formula she said she compounded for the Queen of Sheba:

Queen of Sheba's Super Sex Tonic

Take: one-quarter cup fresh cabbage juice
one-quarter cup fresh carrot juice
one-quarter cup fresh potato juice
one-half teaspoonful crushed
spearmint leaves
one-half teaspoonful crushed
peppermint leaves
one-quarter teaspoonful crushed cloves
one-eighth teaspoonful Ceylon cinnamon
Mix furiously until all of the
ingredients are completely blended.
Drink one cupful
three times a day.

Once again, this is reportedly the formula that the escaped slave made public in a letter which was written during her lifetime but was not to be opened until after her death. We don't know if this was all of the ingredients.

Was she still faithful to the queen and the promise she had made to keep her magic love mixture secret? Will the use of this mixture turn you and your partner into the king and queen of sex?

Give it a shot . . . it can't hurt!

King Henry VIII was no slouch in the bed chamber. His secret is not much of a secret since everyone can find it and use it at any time. It's parsley—the green leafy vegetable on your plate along with the hamburger that you carefully put to one side and then throw out.

Parsley is a member of the celery family. It gained a wide following starting as far back as the 3rd century B.C. when Greece and Rome were in flower. At that time it was not used so much as a vegetable but as an herb that could revitalize tired members.

It began to be considered a vegetable when bored wives began putting the parsley into stews and broths. Their husbands didn't know they were being given an aphrodisiac—they only marvelled at their newfound vigor and vitality.

Some say the use of parsley alarmed the clergy who kept it away from the people until the 10th century. Europe and England did not partake of this herb until parsley plants were introduced secretly into the lands.

The nutritional power is in the leaves with large amounts of vitamins A and C, and the minerals iron, iodine, copper and manganese; plus a unique gland-stimulating oil which is released as the parsley is crushed between the teeth.

Parsley juice is very powerful and if you decide to juice this herb, add only a little bit to a glass of pineapple juice. (Too much causes the heart to race.)

However, the next time you order a hamburger, eat the little green sprigs on the side. It's the most healthful thing on the plate.

Caligula was mad, insane, crazy out of his mind.

But did he begin to go mad because of his wife? Mrs. Caligula (Caesonia) habitually visited the stables when new colts were foaled. Many of them were born with a small bit of extra flesh on the forehead.

Caesonia would remove that bit of flesh, mix it with some of Caligula's blood (she opened a vein), and serve it to him. The mixture was called *hippomanes* and would inflame Caligula to new heights of passion, perhaps even to madness.

Then again, consider the magic potion of Medea of Thessaly who, according to Seneca (Roman dramatist) used the following in her wicked ways:

> *. . . venom extracted from serpents,*
> *entrail and organs of unclean birds,*
> *the heart of a screech owl*
> *and vampire's vitals,*
> *ripped from living flesh.*

This is a story that runs from 1620 until 1705. Ann de Lanclos (*Ninon de Lenclos*) was a French courtesan, known to most of the famous men of her generation like Molière and Scarron. Her life was so filled with scandalous amorous encounters that she was forced into retirement and made to enter a nunnery.

After a period of time she was released to write a book about her life and the famous people she had known. Until her death at age 85 she was still beautiful, still youthful in body and face, her skin was smooth and unwrinkled, and her perfumed garden still moist and functioning . . . so much so that her great-grandson attempted to seduce her. (Did she or didn't she?)

Anyway, she said she owed her youthfulness and her continued sexual appetite and attractiveness to a daily ritual, her bath.

But not just any bath. Her bathwater was fragrant with herbs. This is her secret formula:

Courtesan's Pleasure

Mix together a handful each of the fresh or dried herbs:

lavender flowers
rosemary
mint
crushed comfrey root
thyme
celandine

Put the mixture into an earthenware crock and pour one quart of boiling water over it. Let stand covered for 20 minutes then pour the clear portion into the tub.
Get in and just relax for 15 minutes.

Try daydreaming about your favorite fantasy as you soak and see if you don't feel like fulfilling that scenario after this aromatic beauty bath.

FLOWERS, FRAGRANCES AND ESSENTIAL OILS

For thee the wonder-working earth
puts forth sweet flowers.
Lucretius 99–55 B.C.

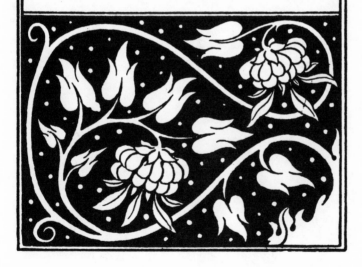

IT'S NO accident that orchid blooms are highly prized, that bringing flowers is a sure way to make a great impression on a first date, that "Say it with flowers" was such a meaningful slogan. Certain flowering plants have age-old meanings attached to them, many related to their aphrodisiacal qualities or status as symbols of fertility. The colors of flowers have also been symbolically linked to special meanings.

The power of fragrances (such as those from flowers) to stir the memory is understood by scientists today. Our sense of smell is not as acute as in centuries gone by due to overbombardment from competing fumes (industry, autos, chemicals, synthetic scents, etc.). Yet most of us can, in the space of a second, recall specific people or scenes through the stimulus of a sudden whiff of a long-since-forgotten odor.

Add to aroma the sense of touch—through massage with a warm, fragrant essential oil—and you have the makings of a truly memorable erotic encounter.

Many people used flowers to create aphrodisiac mixtures. Cakes were baked using purple cyclamens and fed to swains lacking the impetus to yield to love.

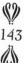

Dr. Edward Bach of Bach Flower Remedies, recommended fuchsia essence to treat sexual inertia while the ancient Greeks considered the morning-glory flower to be able to instill and prolong the love tussle.

Indian doctors prescribe flowers of the ylang-ylang for impotence and frigidity.

Chinese women make soup from the jasmine flower and frequently toss it into tea. Jasmine tea, when sipped at body temperature, can rouse even the most tired of members.

Tahitian girls take the blossoms from the tiara flower and brew a potent mixture they feed to their lover.

Romans in ages past plucked rose leaves and rose blossoms, violet petals, lavender, saffron, rosemary and mixed them with resinous myrrh and honey. But the top spot in flower magic is offered by the ancient Teutons. Germans are not particularly noted for love poetry but this potion is as charming as any poetry in history:

Take the most beautiful flowers of three roses, pink, white, and red and wear them close to your heart for three days. Then, pick a sweet wine blended from red and white and let the roses steep for three more days. Then on three successive nights feed your lover from this magic wine and he will forevermore be yours.

Flowers and floral essences in the bath-water can be very conducive to lovemaking at any age. They can be used prior to intercourse to scent the skin and will not interfere with natural stimulating odors. They make the skin smooth and slippery and more sensitive to the touch. History reports on a number of herbal combinations for different occasions. Here are some for you to try:

Flower Fancy

Take one ounce of each of the following:

vervain	sage
orris root	linden
vetiver	clover
white oak	southernwood

Bring one quart of water to a boil
and add one ounce of the mixed herbs.
Let simmer for five minutes.
Strain and use the clear liquid
in the bathwater.

Waterfall for Two

Take one ounce each of the following:

rose buds	bay leaf
acacia flowers	rosemary
orange buds	myrtle
jasmine flowers	thyme

Add one-half teaspoonful of musk.
Bring one quart of water to a boil
and add one ounce of the mixed herbs.
(Save the rest in an airtight jar
for your next liaison.)
Lower the heat and let simmer
for about 10 minutes.
Then turn off the heat
and half fill your tub with warm water.
Strain the mixture and
pour the clear liquid into the tub.
Add 25 drops of ambergris tincture
and get into the tub.
Then, invite your lover to come
and soak with you.
If this doesn't arouse him
. . . check his pulse.

Although this bath is less fragrant than the above flower formula, some women and most men will react very strongly to the combined odors of bath and body.

Woodsy Wonder Bath

Take one ounce each of:

myrtle	tansy
plantain	linden
oak bark	vervain
orange leaf	benzoin

Put up one quart of water to boil
and add one ounce of the mixed herbs.
Let simmer for 10 minutes.
Strain and
add
the clear liquid to your bath.

Because smell is a variable, some people will react more favorably to one scent mixture over another. So try one combination and if it doesn't have the desired result don't give up . . . try another.

The compelling power of scent on the pysche has been recognized since the earliest of times. Aromatic woods, gums and herbs were burned to drive out "evil spirits" and *kyphi*, an ancient Egyptian perfume, was said to lull to sleep, allay anxieties and brighten dreams. In ancient times and now today, aromatic oils are employed for their soporific, antidepressant or aphrodisiac properties.

In the animal kingdom the female often gives off an aphrodisiac odor when she is ready to mate. Our human society has evolved in such a manner that such advertising is not considered proper or necessary. That's not to say that natural sexual body odors don't play an important part, just that we tend to overlook or downplay their importance in favor of manufactured or borrowed scents.

We do give off arousing scents, not only from the genital area but also in perspiration and from hair and skin. The effects of these aromas are heightened during sexual intercourse.

Plants contain sexy scents they use to attract insects for their mating practices and we humans have appropriated their volatile oils for our mating practices.

Feeling good and feeling sexually aroused are linked, but different. The area of the brain related to the smell response is also linked to a condition known as euphoria. This simply means feeling high or on top of the world. When you feel good you are more easily put into a loving mood. Some of the most effective plant oils that have been known to make people feel good are also the same plant oils that make people feel sexy.

The essential oil obtained from Clary sage, or *Salvia sclarea* is thought to be an aphrodisiac. According to experts, the musky odor of the flowers and of their essential oil justifies their very effective erogenous application. No doubt the euphoric and aphrodisiac qualities are linked in some way. There is some suspicion that it might stimulate the release of adrenaline, and it certainly has some effect on the sex hormones, probably stimulating the release of estrogen.

As early as 1866 Guibourt reported in his *Natural History of Simple Drugs* that ylang-ylang flowers were made into a pomade with coconut oil in the Molucca islands. In the winter it was rubbed into the whole body to guard against fevers and it was used all year round by the young women who perfumed their hair with it after bathing.

Although two M.D.s, Gatti and Cayola, reported the oil to be an aphrodisiac in 1920, the best trial and error was performed by a young lady who gave her best beau a backrub with a little bit of the essence. When questioned, her response was simply, "I'll take another bottle."

If impotence is a problem, eat a good balanced diet, take vitamins and try this mixture of essential oils:

Sizzling Sitz Bath

Into a basin big enough for you to sit in,
put enough tepid water to cover
your genitals when you sit down and:
two drops of pepper essence
five drops of clary sage
two drops of jasmine.
Sit in this mixture for 10 minutes
and see if this has put the lead back
into your pencil.
Repeat in 48 hours if necessary.

Everyone needs an energy refueling now and again. This bath will put the tiger back in your tank and have her purring like a kitten:

Revitalizing Soak

In a tub of warm water, place:
two drops of essence of basil
four drops of essence of geranium
two drops of hyssop
Get in the tub and soak for 20 minutes,
then take a multivitamin and
have a protein meal.

This works when you're in the mood
and he's ready to go to sleep:

Magic Massage Oil

Mix:
six drops of rose essence
four drops of jasmine
four drops of bergamot
eight drops of sandalwood
in 50 cc of vegetable oil.
Begin by massaging yourself until the
aroma, warmed by your body, gets to him.
Then start to massage him.
Let him massage you.
Soon the magic mixture will have
the two of you singing
love's old sweet song.

Buy all of the herbs in the amounts you will need. This mixture is enough for 10 baths:

Super Sex Splash

patchouli, three ounces
geranium leaf, three ounces
mint, two ounces
orange leaf, two ounces
sage, two ounces
strawberry leaf, one ounce
pennyroyal, one ounce
woodruff, one ounce
rosemary, one ounce
Take a handful of the mixture,
place it in an earthenware bowl
and pour a quart of boiling water on it.
Let steep for 20 minutes then pour
the clear liquid into your bath water.
In a flash you'll be ready for sex.

Or maybe your lover prefers showers. No problem.

Prepare your rejuvenating liquid the same way.

Reviving Rub-Down

Strain and put the residue into
the middle of a washcloth.
While he's showering,
rub him down with the washcloth.
Tie the ends of the washcloth together
to make an herbal bag and
rub his skin gently.
Then use the liquid as a final rinse.

If he doesn't give you a standing ovation,
ring the neighbor's bell!

But who is this . . . an amber scent of odorous
  perfume
Her harbinger?   John Milton 1608–1674

This internal method of attraction is called
"The Ultimate Aphrodisiac." Flowers use
it all the time to attract flying creatures
from afar to pick up their pollen and send
it to a neighbor.

Strictly for women, it's the jasmine
douche! It's the court of last and strongest
appeal when nothing else has worked on
your man.

Use with caution . . . and send the kids
to a sitter first.

153

Cupid's Jasmine Douche

one-half cup rosebuds
one-half cup rose hips
one-half cup jasmine flowers
one-half cup regular tea leaves
one drop real (not synthetic)
oil of jasmine
Boil 16 ounces of water in a glass or
earthenware container.
Turn off the heat
and put in one-third cup of this mixture.
Cover and let steep for 10 minutes.
Strain, pour the liquid
into your regular bag,
add enough water to fill the bag
and douche.

The same mixture makes a delightful tea if you add a bit of honey and lemon. After the first encounter has reached its happy conclusion, wait a few minutes then serve tea in bed.

The aroma wafting from both warm, wet sources will soon demand a repeat performance.

And you thought all herbalists were old women with warts, living alone in the forest with only a cat for company, stirring all sorts of nasty things into an iron pot, all the while chanting spells . . .

Now you know they use earthenware pots because iron interferes with the action!

AMBERGRIS

When a human or animal gets sick to the stomach and relieves itself by regurgitating, the resultant is disposed of or avoided as quickly as possible. However, when a whale vomits, the glutinous mass floats on the surface of the ocean to become a prize for whoever is lucky enough to come across it.

Whale vomit is highly prized in the perfume industry because it prolongs the fine odor of the flower and softens its fragrance.

A tiny amount of this substance taken by mouth is said to restore a youthful ability to the aged, and vastly increased sexual power to the virile. According to Boswell, three grains (about enough to cover the tip of the nail on your pinky) could arouse a camel while a gram would drive an elephant wild.

This may be so but I, for one, would rather forgo the pleasures of connubial bliss than take a bite of whale vomit.

SCULLCAP / *Scutellaria lateriflora*

The plant was named such because its blossoms resembled the human skull. It has also been called madweed because it was used against hydrophobia. It was also used for hysteria, St. Vitus dance and convulsions.

Although most uses for herbs were determined by the trial and error method, some herbalists used the "signature method."

According to the Doctrine of Signatures, it was believed that nature had indicated what herbs were useful for what conditions by certain signs. For example, if a plant grew in water this meant it was good for the genito-urinary system. If it grew in a rocky ground it was good against "stones," and so on. The color of the leaves and flowers also were indications for its medicinal use.

Red is the color of blood. It was concluded that plants with red flowers could be useful to the blood. This turns out to be not so farfetched since modern science has found that the red color in the flowers is mostly due to iron which is needed to manufacture hemoglobin. Red clover is one example.

Blue is soothing and sedative. These plants with blue-colored flowers are helpful to nerves and brain disorders. The blue color is due, in part, to the minerals potassium and phosphorus, which are nutrients important to nerve transmission. Valerian, vervain and scullcap are examples.

Yellow suggests the color of bile, so herbs carrying yellow flowers were much in demand for digestive problems, liver problems and gall disorders. Yellow flowers contain sodium which is needed for digestion and liver secretions. Good digestives with yellow blossoms are celandine and barberry.

Scullcap is a great tranquilizer and nervine. If sexual congress makes you nervous and unable to relax enough to really enjoy it, you might try it. It can be mixed with tobacco and smoked for a soothing journey.

Or steep one ounce of the herb in a pint of very hot water for 20 minutes. Strain, add honey and drink a glass or two.

Caution: Because the chemistry of scullcap has not been determined do not mix it with any other tranquilizer.

❧ Essential Oils ❧

The essential oils of certain plants also have been used as aphrodisiacs. Essential oils, also called volatile oils or essences, are the substances that give the aroma to flowers, attract or repel insects, contribute to fertilization, and carry plant hormones.

Most perfumes can be sensual, especially when massaged or applied to body parts; however, the essences can also be used internally when obtained from certain plants. Be sure that the essences you buy are natural essences, because synthetic essences are not to be used internally.

ANISEED / *Pimpinella anisum*

Take four to six drops on a sugar cube twice a day.

CINNAMON / *Cinnamomum zeylanicum*

Drink two to three drops in honey water twice daily.

PEPPERMINT / *Mentha piperita*

Sip two drops in honey water twice a day.

SANDALWOOD / *Santalum album*

Take two to four drops in honey water twice a day.

YLANG-YLANG / *Canangium odoratum*

Place two to five drops in an alcoholic solution or honey water and drink three times a day.

> *The red rose whispers of passion*
> *And the white rose breathes of love.*
> John Boyle O'Reilly 1844–1890

MUSK ROSE / *Rosa maschata*

In India, a particular species of rose is cultivated for its appeal to the senses and actually prescribed to older men as a marital aid. The musk rose is used to prepare a perfume for use by the female desiring to provoke renewed sexual contact with her mate. The flower is also used to scent tea to be taken before the proposed union.

Of course there's nothing in the books that says this rose cannot be used by other than married women to incite their husbands to lust after them. You don't have to sign a declaration of intent when you purchase this perfume. Is it available in the United States?

Maybe.

❦ Orchids of Eros ❦

Why do so many corsages used in weddings feature an orchid?

In Africa, the Zulus chew the root of the orchid *Lissochilus arenarius* and on the stem of *Ansellia gigantea* and swear by its ability to bring on amorous action.

Orchis mascula cooked in a base of wine and chestnuts with pistachios, pine nuts, cinnamon, peppers and sugar appears in *The Witch's Handbook of Love*.

Maybe the groom should forgo the bridal feast and fortify himself by eating the corsage!

Orchis latifolia

Dioscorides mentions that the eating of the roots of this orchid by males causes them to beget male children but if women eat the root when it has dried and withered they shall become like the root . . . barren and withered.

However, if women eat the full root in its prime in a mixture of goat's milk and cinnamon they will engage happily in lustful frolic.

Dendrobium macrael

This is another orchid. The whole plant is used or just the root and the stem.

It is one of the most popular of Indian remedies and a decoction of the whole plant is considered effective for men or women.

LETTER PLANT
Grammatophyllum speciosum

The seeds of this orchid are used in the Solomon Islands in love potions.

PASSIONFLOWER / Passiflora incarnata

Passionflower is a perennial, yellow-flowering vine with a name that has inspired many people to investigate its possibilities.

It contains harmine and other alkaloids and is an MAO inhibitor so take the usual precautions.

Passionflower can be brewed as a tea. The usual method is to take one-quarter ounce of leaves per one pint of water and bring to a boil. Let steep, strain and have a cup.

JASMINE / *Jasminium officinale*

Jasmine flowers calm the nerves but the scent which arises from the volatile oil (essence) arouses erotic interests. If you can afford it, mix two or three drops with some almond oil and massage both bodies.

FINGERLEAF MORNING GLORY
Ipomoea digitata

Taking the powdered root with honey will do the job, as long as the apparatus is functioning.

HONEYSUCKLE / *Lonicera japonica*

The flowers, vines and leaves are said to increase vitality.

APHRODISIACS
THROUGH
THE AGES

The world will always welcome lovers
As time goes by.   *Herman Hupfeld 1894–1951*

ANCIENT peoples—Jews, Romans, Greeks, Chinese—had the same problems and feelings as modern people . . . only more so. We have television, movies, tapes, refrigeration, corner drugstores and lots of water to bathe in.

The sexual impulse, while strong enough, is perhaps more easily satisfied by other pursuits today than it was yesterday. Then, the health of the individual, the balance of his personality, depended on the preservation or the recovery of his sexual potency.

Besides the preservation of the species, it was more important in those days because what else was there to do at night?

So it was no wonder that men sought release from exhaustion due to overindulgence and older men sought to avoid the sexual decline usually brought on by aging.

And it was not only the men who had problems. Women wanted to enjoy sex and wanted to bear young. In those days a woman without the ability to have children was not valued too highly.

So whole cultures sought out the means to invoke more and better sex and means to avoid barrenness. Among the earliest

165

references to aphrodisiacs was this reference in the Old Testament:

And Reuben went in the days of the wheat harvest and found mandrake in the field, and brought them unto his mother Leah. Then Rachel went to Leah, give me, I pray thee, of thy son's mandrake.

Also in the Song of Solomon, Chapter VII, verse 13:

The mandrakes give a smell and at our gates are all manner of pleasant fruits, new and old, which I have laid up for thee, O my beloved.

Not much can be understood from these quotations but Leah did bear a fifth child after the mandrakes and it is shown that the plant was found in the fields at harvest time. So what of the mandrake plant?

It was highly esteemed because of its rarity and for its ability to do two things: influence the ability to conceive and stimulate the ability to copulate.

In the Hebrew language *dudain* has been translated to mean mandrake. Dudain means a fruit with a sweet and agreeable odor which is desired by males. The word

is said to be derived from *Dudim* (the pleasures of love).

Although authorities have translated the
Bible from the original, there is some doubt
whether dudain and mandrake are actually the same. Mandrake is a poisonous
root and not a fruit.

Pythagoras was impressed by the shape
of the root and its resemblance to the human form. It often has an additional root-
let which resembles a penis. He called it
manlikeness root or *mandrake*.

The sexual virtues of the mandrake were
appreciated by the Greeks and Romans as
well. Dioscorides was aware of its reputation and wrote that it was utilized often as
a love potion, increasing sexual desire and
potency, and as an aid to end female
sterility.

It's amazing that nowhere is it written
that women have sexual desires or that
some women would be glad to take aphrodisiacs to stimulate their desires!

Pliny spoke of the mandrake as follows:

*The whole variety of the Eryngium known as
the centum capita in our language has some
marvellous facts recorded of it. It is said to have*

a striking likeness to the organs of generation of either sex; it is rarely met with, but if a root resembling the male organ of the human species be found by a man, it will ensure him woman's love; hence it is said that Phaon, the Lesbian, was so passionately beloved of Sappho . . .

Some people thought there was great danger in the picking of the mandrake root. When plucked from the earth, they believed the root screamed like a soul in agony and the sound was enough to drive the picker into instant insanity.

Shakespeare refers to it in *Romeo and Juliet*, Act IV, scene three:

And shrieks like mandrakes torn out of the earth,
That living mortals, hearing them, run mad.

But what is the mandrake actually? Can it live up to its legend?

Actually, it's a member of the potato family, named *Mandragora officinarium* by less imaginative scientists. It is found chiefly in the Mediterranean regions and has a thick root frequently forked to look like two legs. The fruit is orange in color and resembles fleshy berries. It was used medicinally for its narcotic actions, but is no longer considered to be effective for that purpose.

Later superstition has it that the mandrake springs up at the foot of the gallows. This is why: A man who is hanged was thought, during the death agony, to experience erection and ejaculation. The sperm fell to earth and the mandrake was born, legend has it.

Ever since, the mandrake and its connection with sexuality was frozen in folklore.

More famous than mandrake is the *satyrion* of Greece and Rome. Although it is not certain exactly what satyrion was, it appears to be some kind of orchid. The Arab *sahlab* (salep) may have a connection with satyrion. Salep is a medicine herb used in the Orient as a nervine and restorative. The roots of various species of orchid are washed and the outer layer is removed. Then they are heated until they assume a horny appearance and dried slowly.

Plutarch in his *De Sanitate tuenda* wrote of satyrion as producing a stimulating effect. Dioscorides and Pliny wrote that the root will produce excitement if merely carried in the hand.

Petronius, in his *Satyricon,* mentions:

Accordingly we followed the pair, who led us along the name-boards, where we saw in the chambers persons of both sexes behaving in such a fashion I concluded they must every one have been drinking satyricon . . .

Some say the basis of these satyricon potions was the root of the *orchis-hircina.* This was dissolved in goat's milk and "given to exhausted old men to rekindle within them the fires of love."

It was said that Hercules, after being given the potion by Thespius, deflowered the 50 daughters of his hostess, requiring just one night to complete the labors of love.

Proculus, after drinking liberally of the potion, "turned 100 virgin prisoners into women in only 15 days," that comes to less than seven a day . . . nothing compared to Hercules.

It seems likely that something like hashish was mixed in the potion to produce such tales of potency. Even if they happened, and it's likely that something did happen, it's probable they were exaggerated as the years went by.

Many other means of achieving erection and curing impotence were known to Greeks and Romans. One of the preparations contained powdered peppers mixed with the seeds from the nettle plant. Others combined onions, wild cabbage, eggs, honey and pineapple. Another popular potion contained feverfew, pellitory and old wine.

The pith from the pomegranate tree (*Punica granatum*) was believed able to increase sexual potency, particularly in combination with the testicles of the ass, an animal of considerable amorous propensity.

Mushrooms, birthworts, and resins were happily recommended, but exact recipes were closely guarded.

Horace cites rockets (beans) as incitants to lust, and savory is mentioned in combination. Colewort (*Eruca*) was said to be a salacious herb sacred to the god Priapus.

⚜ Scentual Seduction ⚜

Ancient Romans devoted a lot of attention to the value of the diet and amatory prowess. What was eaten during the day contributed greatly to the power of the night. In addition, Romans counted heavily on the use of scents. Musk, civet, ambergris and other stimulating perfumes were worn in their hair, on their clothes and sprinkled on their bodies and their bedclothes. Breath was sweetened with spices. Unlike the ancient Greeks and Arabs, the Romans were intensely aware of odors.

A legendary aphrodisiac herb called moly was mentioned by Latin writers as having considerable magic powers. Homer said it was given to Ulysses by Hermes as a protection against the enchantments of Circe. It had a black root with white flowers. The term moly is also applied to *Allium moly* or wild garlic. However, in this modern day, it is uncertain what plant is the legendary moly.

Some say it is *Peganum harmala*, a plant from which the stimulating alkaloid harmaline can be extracted. However, flowers of this plant are white with green stripes so the description does not match Homer's.

Tennyson, in his *Lotus Eaters* speaks of ". . . beds of amaranth and moly."

The ancient Arabs were a little more exact in their writings of aphrodisiacs and other means of increasing physical pleasures.

The Perfumed Garden for the Soul's Delectation was translated from the Arabic of the Sheik Nefzawi by Sir R.F. Burton in 1907.

This was the most popular book in Europe for a time, revealing for the first time Arabic amatory practices. The first of the recipes reads as follows:

"If you want to acquire strength for coitus, take fruit of the mastic tree, pound them well and macerate them with oil and honey, then drink of this first thing in the morning: This will produce an abundance of sperm and make you vigorous."

The second says if you want the same result, "Rub the virile member . . . with gall from the jackal. The rubbing stimulates these parts and increases their vigor."

Other recipes include drinking a glass of honey, 20 almonds and 100 grains of the pine tree. This must be done for three days. Then pound onion seed, sift it and mix it afterward with honey, and take the mixture while fasting.

Cubeb pepper (*Piper cubeba*) is mentioned in passing. A little of it is to be chewed and swallowed with a lot of saliva. Alternatively cardamom grains may also be chewed. Several ancient authors mention the value of rubbing the cardamom-mixed saliva over the glans of the member. Ointment prepared from the *Balm of Judea* employed in the same way is said to produce pleasant effects.

Another recipe from Nefzawi is:

"Pound very carefully together *Anthemis pyrethrum* with ginger, mix them while pounding with an ointment of lilac, then rub this compound into your abdomen, your testicles, and the verge. This will make you ardent." (Lilac ointment was prepared from lilac leaves and oil or fat.)

To relieve impotence:

"You must take galanga (*Galanga major*), cinnamon from Mecca, cloves, Indian cachou (Indian *harchar*), nutmeg, Indian cubebs, sparrow wort (*Stallens panerina*) pyrether, laurel seed and gilly-flowers. Pound all of these together and mix in pigeon broth (chicken broth can be used instead). You must drink as much as you can morning and night. Drink water before and after the broth."

For premature ejaculation:

"Mix nutmeg and oliban with honey. Tablespoon of the mixture is to be taken three times daily on an empty stomach."

A second potion for relief of premature ejaculation is:

Take the following in honey: pyrether, nettleseed, spurge, cedaville, ginger, cinnamon, caraway, cardamom, and mix ginger with more honey. Said mixture is to be rubbed into the surface of the member after it has been washed lightly in tepid water and gently rubbed dry.

Ancient Passion Potions

Many other potent combinations are offered in this titillating book:

"Camel's milk mixed with honey and taken regularly . . . causes the virile member to be alert night and day."

"He who for several days makes his meals upon eggs boiled with myrrh, coarse cinnamon and pepper, will find his vigour . . . greatly increased."

"Take one part of the juice pressed out of pounded onions, and mix it with two parts of purified honey. Heat the mixture over a fire until the onion juice has disappeared and the honey only remains. Then take the residue from the fire, let it cool, and preserve it for use when wanted. Then mix 12 drams of it with three pints of water, and let chick peas be macerated in this fluid for one day and one night.

"This beverage is to be taken of during winter and on going to bed. Only a small quantity is to be taken, and only for one day. The member of him who has drunk of it will not give him much rest during the night that follows."

The Perfumed Garden also teaches, for the first time in Arab lands, the science of perfumes and love:

"The use of perfumery by men should be included amongst those things which conduce the sexual union; for when as the women doth inhale the odour of the scent she waxeth faint and shortly becomes utterly distraught. Yea oft times have men been assisted in obtaining possession of women through the seductive influence of the odour of those perfumes with which they had previously been at pains to besprinkle themselves . . ."

The Arabs believe that four parts of the body should be perfumed: the mouth, the nose, the armpits, and the pudenda.

Abu Ali al-Husain ibn Sina, a physician, has written much about coital technique.

Among his remedies for increasing pleasure are: The taking of cubeb into the
mouth and honey with scammony; also
ginger with pepper is chewed and the saliva applied to the end of the penis, a
procedure that may result in an unpleasant
irritation, but reportedly increases the size
of the penis.

A pharmaceutical firm in London, in 1943
and maybe even until now, made and was
selling a cream for penile application based
on an old Arab formulation. It was sold
with the claim that it delayed orgasm and
increased rigidity.

A rather recent sage of amour was Omar
Haleby, who gives us the following recipe:

"Take 15 grams of aromatic leaves of
stoechas and of saffron; 20 of anise and
wild carrot; 25 pieces of orange blossoms;
50 dried dates; 4 pieces of egg-yolk; 500
grams of clear water.

"Boil the whole for half an hour in an
earthen-covered pot. Then remove it from
the fire and stir slowly.

"Next add 50 grams of honey and the fresh
blood of two doves. Let it remain for 24
hours, during which time it should be stirred
several times. Finally pass it through a sieve.

"For one week take one or two tea-spoonfuls half an hour before retiring, and before every coition."

Moroccans employ an electuary called madchun. This is composed of honey, acorns, various nuts, sweet almonds, butter, flour, sesame, hashish and cantharides. The last ingredient is extremely dangerous even if it is surrounded by a variety of nutritional foods. Its vesicant action as it enters the genito-urinary area can cause severe irritation to the point of internal bleeding. However, the user was aware of the risk . . . presumably!

Mention is also made of a Moroccan root called surnag said to increase potency.

In Constantinople, little pastilles were used. These were made from hemp buds (*Cannabis indica*), honey, muscat nuts and saffron.

Another preparation was made from *Cannabis indica*, carnations, moschus, coconut and honey.

Henna was also held in high esteem as a means of curing inorganic male impotence. It was said that rubbing henna on the fingertips, the skull and the sternum, proved to be a natural cure. In extreme cases henna was also applied to the soles of the feet.

Henna is well known as a hair dye. It's prepared by gathering the leaves and young twigs and grinding them to a fine powder. As a drug, it can restrain perspiration in the hands and feet when rubbed on these parts. It produces an agreeable coolness conducive to health and comfort.

The Turkish people have faith in perfumery as being among the best adjuvants to aiding sexual desire and potency. One of their formulas is compounded as follows:
Take:

olibanum (frankincense)	2.5 grams
rosewater	500.0 grams
musk	50.0 grams
myrrh	50.0 grams
camphor	50.0 grams

Thoroughly powder this combination and place into a glass jar which is then hermetically sealed. Place the jar where it will receive sunlight and leave for 48 hours.

Afterwards it is gradually clarified, altered, and kept in a suitable receptacle. To insure its staying power, add 75 grams of rectifying alcohol and three drops of Essence of Baghdad Rose.

A small spoonful is added to the washing water; it is sprayed on clothing, or applied in other usual fashions.

It is said that this scintillating scent "affects the brain, the heart, the genitals, and the consciousness."

India also had a great affection for scents but used them often in a different manner. A fine powder was made from *Tabernamontana coronaria* and *Flacourtia cataphracts*. This was then applied to the wick of a lamp and burned softly into the air.

How about these ancient Indian methods employed to "subjugate a woman to one's will":

"If a man, after anointing his lingam with a mixture of the powders of the white thorn apple, the long pepper, and the black pepper and honey, engages in sexual union with a woman, he makes her subject to his will.

"The application of a mixture of the leaf of the plant *Vatodbhranta*, of the flowers thrown on a human corpse when carried out to be burned, and the powder of the bones of the peacock, and of the jiwanjiva bird produces the same effect.

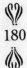

"The remains of a kite (hawk) who has died a natural death, ground into a powder, and mixed with cowach and honey, has also the same effect.

"If pieces of arris root are dressed with the oil of the mango, and placed for six months in a hole made in the trunk of the sisu tree, and are taken out and made up as an ointment, and applied to the lingam, this is said to serve as the means of subjugating women . . ."

More practical are these means of increasing sexual vigor:

♡ A man gains sexual vigor by drinking milk mixed with sugar, the root of the uchchata plant, the piper chaba and licorice.

♡ Drinking milk with sugar is good but having the testicle of a ram or goat boiled in it is better.

♡ The seed of the long pepper along with the seeds of the *Sanseviera roxburghiana* and the *Hedysarum gangeticum* plant, all pounded together and mixed with milk, will help to renew sexual strength.

♡ If a man pounds the seeds or roots of the trapa bispinosa, the kasurika, the tuscan jasmine, and licorice, together with the kshirakapoli (a kind of onion) and puts the powder into milk mixed with sugar and ghee (clarified butter), and having boiled the whole mixture on a moderate fire, drinks the paste so formed, he will be able to enjoy innumerable women.

♡ If a man takes the outer covering of sesamum seeds, and soaks them with the eggs of the sparrow, and then, having boiled them with milk, mixed with sugar and ghee, along with the fruits of the trapa bispinosa and the kasurika plant, and adding to it the flour of wheat and beans, and then drinks of this composition, he is said to be able to enjoy many women.

♡ If ghee, honey, sugar and licorice in equal quantities, the juice of the fennel plant, and milk are mixed together, this nectar-like composition is said to be holy, and provocative of sexual vigor, a preservative of life and sweet to the taste.

♡ The drinking of a paste composed of the asparagus racemosus, the shvadaustra plant, the goduchi plant, the long pepper, and licorice, boiled in milk, honey, and ghee, in the spring is said to have the same effect.

♡ Boiling the asparagus racemosus, and

the shvadaustra plant, along with the pounded fruits of the premna spinosa in water, and drinking the water is said to act in the same way.

On enlarging the *lingam* (after a phallic symbol used in Hindu worship):
"When a man wishes to enlarge his lingam, he should rub it with the bristles of certain insects and then, after rubbing it for 10 nights with oils, he should then rub it with bristles as before. By continuing to do this a swelling will be gradually produced in the lingam . . ."
After this he should take away all the pain and swelling by using cool concoctions. The swelling is called *ʃuka* and is often brought about among the Dravidians of Southern India.
(This should not be attempted by anyone under any circumstances since it entails severe risks and grave dangers for anyone foolhardy enough to make such a trial.)
Another formula for the same effect:
If the lingam is rubbed with the following things, the plant physalis flexuosa, the shavara-kandaka plant, the jalasuka plant,

the fruit of the eggplant, the butter of the she buffalo, the hastri-charma plant, and the juice of the vajrarasa plant, a swelling lasting for one month (!) will be produced.

Ananga-Ranga or the *Hindu Art of Love* has been translated from the Sanskrit. This volume outdoes the Nefzawi and Vatsyayana in listing 33 subjects including: hastening the paroxysm of the woman; delaying the orgasm of the man; aphrodisiacs; thickening and enlarging the lingam rendering it sound and strong, hard and lusty; "purifying the womb;" causing pregnancy and preventing miscarriage.

Other subjects addressed for eager readers are: clearing the skin of eruptions; enlarging the breasts and raising and hardening pendulous breasts; for giving a fragrance to the skin; for removing the "evil savour" of perspiration; and recipes to enable a woman to attract and preserve her husband's love. (Looking over the 33 subjects it appears that we haven't changed much over the centuries.)

The first recipe: Take some aniseed (*Pimpinella anisum*) reduced to a fine powder and from it make an electuary by softening it with honey. Through application of this paste to the lingam prior to intercourse you will be able to produce orgasm in the woman and she will submit to your will.

The second chapter instructs: Take some rui seed (*Calloptropis gigantea*) and pound thoroughly with the leaves of the jai (*Jasminum auriculatum*) until the juice or essence is expelled from them. Soften and apply as in the previous recipe.

The third deals with premature ejaculation:

Take the root of the Kang (*Panicum italicum*) and the pollen of the lotus flower, pulverize them in honey, and apply the composition to the soles of the feet. The embrace will thus be prolonged by retention of the vital liquor. (Note: The concept of applying substances to the soles of the feet is not so farfetched. People who could not stand the taste of garlic but appreciated the activity of the herb put cloves of it in their shoes. As they walked the pressure released the oil from the garlic which was then absorbed through the skin. Once absorbed, it was circulated throughout the body through the bloodstream.)

After that is written some formulas concerning aphrodisiacs:

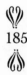

Expose the juice of Bhuya-Kokali (*Solanum jacquini*) under the heat of the sun until it dries, and then mix it with ghee and honey. This preparation gives the strength of 10 men, and enables but one man to satisfy 10 women.

Take the outside covering of the anvalli (*Myrobolan emblica*), an astringent nut *Phyllanthus emblica*, extract the juice and leave in the sun until dry. After this it should be mixed with powder from the same tree, and before congress, eaten with ghee, candied sugar and honey.

From this results a prodigious development of the genital; "even an old man will become like a young one."

Soak urid seeds (*Phaseolus radiata* or *Phaseolus mungo*) in milk and sugar, and expose the mixture for three days to the rays of the sun, reduce to a powder or pasty consistency, knead into the form of cakes and fry in ghee.

This should be eaten each morning and the patient no matter what his age will regain extreme vigour and will be able to enjoy 100 women.

Take 150 grains of the pith of the moh tree *Bassia latifolia* (the flowers of which contain a spirituous liquor well known), pound well in a mortar, and drink after having mixed the powder with the milk of the cow. The effect will be the same as that produced by the recipe immediately preceding.

Weak erections and small members are the next subject. Here are two examples:

Take equal parts of chikana (*Hedysarum lagopodiodes*), lechi, kosth (*Costus speciosus* or *arabicus*), iris root, *Pothos officinalis*, *Physalis flexuosa*, and oleander. Pound these and mix with butter. Apply thin compositions to the organ, and after about "two ghari" (45 minutes) it will attain the largeness of the member of a horse.

For a Long Love Life . . .

Of course, we don't expect you to try any of these preceding wilder recipes from the past, but it's interesting to know how cultures of long ago coped with what they considered their shortcomings.

Today we know that, short of a prosthetic appliance, what you see is what you've got and you've got to learn how to use it.

The best recipe for a great love life is the same as that for a long life—eat a healthy, nutritional diet; don't smoke; don't drink to excess, if at all; and fall in love with the right person. Avoiding unnecessary stress and getting regular exercise is also a good adjunct to any plan for boosting your sex life.

BIBLIOGRAPHY

AURAND, S.H. *Botanical Materia Medica and Pharmacology.* 1899.

CLARKE, J.H. *Dictionary of Practical Materia Medica.* Edinburgh: 1962.

COXE, J.R. *American Dispensatory*, 4th Edition. Philadelphia: 1818.

DAVENPORT, J. *Aphrodisiacs and Love Stimulants.* New York: Lyle Stuart, Inc. 1966.

ELLIS, A. *The Folklore of Sex.* New York: Boni, 1951.

FINCH, B. *Passport to Paradise.* New York: Philosophical Library, 1960.

GUILFOYLE, W.R. *Australian Botany.* 1884.

HIRSCHFIELD, M. *Sexual Customs in the Far East.* New York: Putnam, 1935.

HOOPER, D. *Chinese Medicine*, Vol. VI. 1929.

LEYEL, C.F. *The Magic of Herbs.* 1926.

MACLEOD, D. *A Book of Herbs.* London: 1968.

MILLER, A.M. *The Magical and Ritual Use of Herbs.* New York: Destiny Books, 1983.

OCHSE, J.J. *Vegetables of the Dutch East Indies.* 1931.

POTTER, O.L. *Materia Medica.* London: 1911.

SANYAL, D. and GHOSE, R. *Vegetable Drugs of India.* 1934.

THOMPSON, S.J.S. *The Mystic Mandrake*. London: Rider & Co. 1934.

WALTON, A.H. *Aphrodisiacs from Legend to Prescription*. Westport, Connecticut: Associated Booksellers, 1958.

INDEX

INDEX

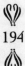

INDEX